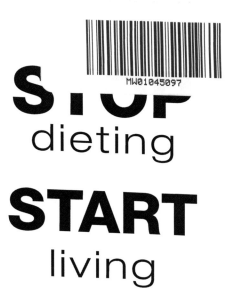

# STOP
## dieting

# START
## living

# STOP
## dieting
# START
## living

A Balanced

Approach to

Health and

Fitness

## Barbara Godfrey

ATE PUBLISHING & Enterprises

Published by Tate Publishing & Enterprises, LLC
127 E. Trade Center Terrace | Mustang, Oklahoma 73064 USA
1.888.361.9473 | www.tatepublishing.com

Tate Publishing is committed to excellence in the publishing industry. The co reflects the philosophy established by the founders, based on Psalm 68:11,
*"The Lord gave the word and great was the company of those who published*

Book design copyright © 2010 by Tate Publishing, LLC. All rights reserved.
*Cover design by Amber Lee*
*Interior design by Jeff Fisher*

Published in the United States of America

ISBN: 978-1-60799-088-8
1. Health & Fitness, Exercise
2. Health & Fitness, Nutrition
10.06.03

# DEDICATION

This book is dedicated to my loving and supportive family and friends, who always believe in everything I do, especially my three boys, Garrett, Austin, and Parker, who inspire me every day to be the best I can be and for appreciating everything I do for them and for adapting to the healthy lifestyle I have taught them to live by. They are living proof that our children will follow the lifestyles we lead! What a reward this has been to see their accomplishments related to their healthy eating and dedication to their training and workouts. I am truly blessed to have such wonderful kids! I also cannot thank my mom, Nethe (a.k.a. Yiaya) enough! With everything I have been through this last year, I could not have survived without you. You have seriously been my rock through my divorce and all of life's challenges and changes! I love you, Mom, more than you will ever know!

# ACKNOWLEDGMENTS

I want to thank everyone in my family for the love and support they always give me. I especially want to thank Shannan Mingo, one of my best friends, for all of her support, love, encouragement, and many dedicated hours she spent working with me to help me accomplish my dream of writing this book. And especially Gary for believing in me, working with me for months on end to finalize this book, and teaching me that patience is the key to success! Without both of them, this would not have happened!

# TABLE OF CONTENTS

# INTRODUCTION

Congratulations! You are on your way to a healthier and happier life. By purchasing my book, you are telling yourself that you are ready for change, and my goal is to help you get there. Have you ever thought of how you would feel being healthy and looking the way you want to look? Now is the time to do it, and I can help you change your life for the better!

We live in a fast-paced world. This pace has affected our lives in ways I don't think we will truly understand until it is too late. We communicate electronically instead of through live conversation; we opt for quick-fix, premade meals for our families because of the perceived time it will save us; we have no time to squeeze in thirty-minute runs with our dogs, so we investigate all kinds of crazy ways to lose weight and deprive our bodies of the nutrition we need. We also spend more money on diet aids than on any other product (*Forbes Magazine,* April 13, 2005). I made the choice not to follow the masses and make the change to improve my life, and I hope you will too.

I was a professional model for several years and traveled all over the world. I saw it all, the creative ways people tried to stay thin. It's not only dangerous but can be life threatening. It was so sad to see what great lengths people would go to look thin. As I am getting older, I can see and feel the pressures I never felt before.

It is difficult to understand. I am in shape. I eat well and have a healthy lifestyle with a happy and healthy family. I felt like something was missing. My kids were at school all day, and I realized I was not as busy as I was used to. I wanted to go to work and had no idea what to do. I have many interests and have worn many hats in my life.

Looking back on my life, I realized what a positive impact my workouts, the way I eat, and my general discipline have had on how I feel as a person. Then I realized I needed to do something I love. I love working out, and I love helping people. People often ask me how I stay in shape and what I eat to look the way I do at my age after three kids.

I decided it was time to put it down on paper and try to help anyone I can to live a healthier life. In the process of writing the book, I continued to do fitness modeling, which then opened another door to my latest endeavor, which was opening a sports nutrition and weight loss store, Nutrishop, in Ladera Ranch, California. All of this has been so rewarding to me to be able to help people, like you, reach the goals they never thought they could!

Making the choice to change your lifestyle to get in shape and eat right can be tough. We all know the bad foods versus the good foods to a certain extent. Yet most people will make every excuse possible to not have to do the work. What you don't realize is that once you make that lifestyle change, it won't be work at all! It will become a habit to eat right and exercise. You will start to feel and see the benefits, which will then help keep you on course to a better life! The benefits outweigh junk food any day! I love the way I feel when I eat really well and exercise regularly. If I don't, I feel terrible and start to feel like I am getting sick and rundown. If I am not consistent in my eating habits, it affects my mood, my energy, my skin, and I just don't feel like working out. I just feel like crap! It's really not worth it to me. Once you get to the point where you really feel good about how you look and feel, you won't crave the bad-for-you foods. You will be so motivated that it just won't be worth it to cheat and eat a bag of cookies or chips. You'll want to just keep going down the right path to health and fitness.

It is so rewarding. Stay with it, and feel the benefits to come! You'll be so grateful you did!

Remember, I am just like you. I am a busy mom with kids and lead a hectic life. I *chose* to *Stop Dieting and Start Living* so I could live my life to the fullest and be the best role model I could be for my kids. The excuses are out there. Now it is time to take control and put your priorities in order.

Would you rather eat what you want or be healthy and look and feel the way you want? Remember, we do have choices. Are you ready to make a change?

# AGE, ATTITUDE, AND EXERCISE

If you are like me, you want to feel, look, and stay young forever! Although it is impossible to stop the normal aging process, we do have some control over aging in general. We can decide to reach our ideal goals of weight, healthy eating and living, and in return delay the degenerative diseases of aging by avoiding the bad habits that accelerate the normal aging process. Some of these bad habits include lack of exercise, poor nutrition, unnecessary drugs or synthetic supplements, alcohol, artificial sweeteners, food dyes, sugar, too much caffeine, lack of sleep, tobacco use, and stress. Sound familiar? We can all relate to this list. Sadly it's how most of us live! It's now our choice to decide if we want to add years to our life or deduct them! It's never too late to change your eating and exercise habits; you are never too old to choose to live a healthy lifestyle! Deciding to make the choice to eat well and exercise might take some time. But don't delay it any longer! Don't let a health scare motivate you. In some cases, however, it may take extreme circumstances to wake people up and cause them to see that they need to get in shape and live a better life, not only for themselves but also for their families. Don't wait for something drastic to happen in your life to make changes for the better. Do it for *yourself* first before your unhappiness with yourself ruins various aspects of your life. What we do to our bodies today is what we will be dealing with tomorrow, be it good or bad! Cancer and disease don't just happen. It takes years to manifest and destroy our bodies. Make the lifestyle change now. Pave the way to a better future of health and well-being!

It's sad to say, but people are spending billions of dollars trying to make themselves look better in superficial ways, always looking for the easy way out. When people come into my store, they most likely want the quick fix, the fat burners! Sure, these products work, but only if you continuously take them. What people do not realize is that you *have* to change your lifestyle and start to pay attention to what you eat and when you eat certain foods. There is no quick fix in life! I look around and see so many people making the choices to get liposuction, hair implants, and hair extensions—all of which are extremely costly. I know most women would much rather be with guys who are in great shape, confident, and might be bald compared to a guy who is fat and insecure but has a full head of hair! It's much more important to be healthy than to be obsessed with the way we look. A healthy lifestyle is about more than eating well and exercising; it's about accepting and embracing your body and treating it well. It's not about waiting until you've reached some ideal weight or some particular goal before learning to notice what's good about yourself and your body. After all, staying motivated requires that we celebrate every success. Maybe your clothes feel a little looser or you're feeling better about the way you look. It's important to notice the steps along the way. The main focus is health, not appearance! Think about it! Yet people spend thousands of dollars on hair treatments and diet aids that don't work. They complain that healthy food is too expensive and joining a gym is too costly and so on. What most people don't realize is that most of our increased healthcare costs are due to the fact that people don't care or pay attention to what they eat or do. It's always the easy way in life that looks most appealing yet can be the most damaging. Diseases will thrive within a poor diet. If we are not taking in the proper vitamins and nutrients, our bodies cannot fight off anything. Our immune systems will break down, and we will get sick. Yet people don't spend the time or money to invest in a healthy lifestyle. Look at how much people spend on health care, especially if they are out of shape or obese. Medical problems will result from both! Heart disease, lung disease, diabetes, and cancer have all been attributed to what we do and do not put in our bodies. If we would just stop and realize the truth that is staring right at us, it would make this whole diet craze go away! With the health care costs continuing to rise, a lot of us can't even afford to have insurance at all. This is all happening because our poor health is getting out of control. The healthcare industry can't keep up with how unhealthy we are. Let's make a change! Are you spending money on diet aids that don't work? Stop and change your way of life instead! It's cheaper, and the benefits outweigh any diet aid out there.

According to the Centers for Disease Control, studies have shown that lupus, colitis, Crohn's disease, and fibromyalgia are all caused by inflammation of the connective tissues. The inflammations are most often caused by increased toxicity and increased acidity in the body caused by unnatural diets and lifestyles. When you cleanse and detoxify your body, the toxins are eliminated and the connective tissues are no longer irritated, and most likely you will no longer experience these symptoms. It can be as simple as adding fruits and vegetables to your diet. Very few of us get our daily recommended amount of fruits and vegetables. It's important to watch what we eat today, as it will be what our tomorrow brings in the means of our health. This is something we all need to be more diligent about and make sure we are eating enough fruits and vegetables. Since our produce is picked before it is ripened on the vine, we are not getting all of the nutrients we should from what we are eating. Because of this, it is extremely important to supplement your body with safe, healthy alternatives. You can find powdered greens and fruits at most health food stores everywhere. Take advantage of this convenience and supply your body with the nutrients it needs. (See the "What and How to Eat" section for suggestions.)

I think as we get older, we are wiser and have been through more life-changing experiences. So we might choose to live the better life of health and fitness because we can see and feel the difference it makes when we do. No matter what your age, it's time to look at yourself and ask if you are doing everything in your power to make yourself the best you can be. Don't make the excuses!

Attitude is everything in life. A good attitude creates good things. People like to be around positive, happy people. If you surround yourself with negativity, negative things will come your way. Make a change in your attitude now. Tell yourself every day when you wake up that you have two choices: either to be in a good mood or in a bad mood. Each time something bad happens, you can choose to be the victim or you can choose to learn from it. Tell yourself that you are worth it and be a better person for your family and friends by taking care of yourself. Then you will only bring good in your life. You will make the right choices to improve yourself and your family.

Don't be the negative person in the room. It is simply exhausting to be around those people. When people talk badly about other people, they usually are talking about themselves. You do not want to be that person. A bad attitude attracts bad things. I always try to make the conscious effort to stay away from people or places that bring me down. You are in charge of your own choices in life, so make the right ones! God has a plan for you, but you have choices along the way, and you have to be healthy enough, physically and spiritually, to carry his plan out. It is up to you to decide what will happen next. With a good attitude, you will want to be healthy and in shape, and everything else will follow.

Feel good about the body and life God gave you. We are all different. No two people are ever going to be the same. Yet we continuously compare ourselves to others. Does this sound familiar? You just finished a workout, you feel great, and you have been doing everything right. You are in the changing room at the gym, and a perfect-looking girl walks in, and now you feel terrible about yourself. You think that if you never got off that treadmill your whole life, you still would never look like her. Women usually are so busy sizing each other up that they forget to remember to look at their own assets. Be positive, and do your best to avoid this kind of behavior. Learn to appreciate what you have and who you are. It isn't about how good we look but how good we *feel.* That is so much more important in life. Always try to remember to make the right choices. You will love the way you feel when you eat healthy and exercise regularly. We all know how we feel when we eat poorly and don't exercise. I see in my store everyday people who come in complaining that they are overweight and have no energy. What I find out is that these people are starving themselves and actually making themselves fatter! If you do not feed your body properly, it will automatically burn muscle for energy. You want to stop that process and eat right so your body will use its best form of energy, which comes from fat! We all want to lose the fat, so eat, and eat right! If I don't eat enough, blood sugar levels drop, and then I just crave terrible food, which puts me in a really bad mood. It's just not worth it! I make sure I always have something healthy on hand to eat to make sure I keep my metabolism going.

In today's society, there is huge pressure to be model-thin and look perfect. However, the focus must be on health and living a moderate lifestyle. This doesn't mean we won't think about what we look like. A lean person is certainly healthier and will have the energy to live a longer life. *Lean* means having a low to average body fat for your body type. This does *not* mean skinny and undernourished. Scales cannot tell you how lean you are.

This is confusing to the person who tries crash diets and his or her weight, therefore acts like a yo-yo. You can lower your weight on the scales by going on those "diets" that only cause you to lose water weight and muscle rather than fat. You will weigh less and maybe wear a smaller size for a while, but you won't be any *leaner,* and the second you go back to your old eating habits, which always happens if you do not make a lifestyle change, you will gain the weight back plus *more*. Diets that promote or promise drastic weight loss are very misleading. When you start a diet, you can potentially drop a lot of weight during the first two weeks. However, if you lose more than two pounds per week, you are losing muscle mass and your metabolism will slow down in response. It's just not worth it! We want to keep that muscle. The more muscle we have, the more fat we burn. It is essential we get enough protein on a daily basis. Protein is a micronutrient that's critical during weight loss. Protein helps maintain lean muscle mass, your blood sugar levels, and your metabolism. Losing weight takes focus and effort. If it sounds too good to be true, it always is!

Genetics *do* play a role in how a body looks. There is nothing we can do about that. However, everyone, no matter his or her genetics, can be lean with dedication and some work. Some genes make this process easier for some people, but we can all achieve this goal of being lean and healthy if we try.

I often hear people use the excuse that the reason they are fat is that they were born with slow metabolisms. Well, you can change that too. Picture yourself as a bonfire. To keep that fire roaring all day, you need to add wood on an ongoing basis. This is true with your body as well. If you feed yourself five to six small meals a day, you are feeding that bonfire throughout the day, and it continues to burn—calories, that is. If you have muscle, you burn even more. Remember, the more muscle you have, the more fat you will burn doing nothing. Get to the gym and lift those weights; build even more muscle!

All day long I hear women say they don't want to lift weights because they are afraid of getting big. Well, let me tell you, you are only going to get bigger than you are right now if you don't have muscle as you age. Lifting weights also helps build your bone density, which we all need as we get older. It is so important to start now. Lifting weights is even

STOP DIETING, START LIVING

more important than cardio. When a person does too much cardio, he or she will burn muscle, not fat. Don't get me wrong; you still need to do cardio! Make the choice to be an active person who will then generally burn more fat than one who is sedentary.

It really *is* so simple. We gain weight by taking in more calories than we burn. So keep track of yourself and burn more calories than you take in. Simple! You can stay in shape, stay lean, and stay healthy by programming your body to be a fat-burning machine by eating small meals that are high in fiber, high in protein, low in fat, and exercising more.

## Barbara's Tips for Staying Active and Positive

- Focus on daily behavior.

- Don't sit and watch TV. Move!

- Find ways that motivate you! I love music, so I turn the music up and get my chores done. It motivates me and puts me in a great mood!

- Set realistic goals.

- Stop thinking of ways you are failing and think of things to do to fix the situation!

- If you work, find ways to get in every bit of exercise when you can. Walk at lunch; take the stairs when you can. Find that parking place far away, not right in front. Every little bit of extra exercise makes the world of difference!

# GETTING MOTIVATED

Knowing what you are striving for is a good way to begin. This knowledge will also come in handy down the road when you are setting goals, measuring your progress, and trying to get motivated again after a setback.

When we are children, one of the first things we are taught is to respect and love others. People forget that we need to love and respect ourselves first. We cannot love others if we do not know how to love ourselves. When you overeat or eat unhealthy foods, are you really doing what is best for you? Show some love and respect for yourself and feed your body with good, clean food. You will be amazed how happy you will be and how good you will feel, and your body will thank you too.

Find the best ways to motivate yourself. Think of things that make you happy. Think of your real internal motivation for losing weight or becoming fit. Is it so you can have the energy to keep up with your kids or so you feel sexy with your spouse or significant other? Then think of the things that make your heart sing, that you really enjoy. Do you enjoy a certain type of music, or do you like to read? Incorporate these into your everyday workouts and meditate or pray that you will remain focused on your real, internal motivation for wanting to do this.

Music really motivates me. I can be tired and walk into the gym and put my iPod on, and I am suddenly full of energy and ready to go. Different songs can make me run faster and maybe remind me of something that makes me happy, so I keep going.

I have been on a run before and did not realize how much time had gone by because I was so into the music. When I first tried a spin class, I was thinking there was no way I would finish! I ended up doing so with ease because I was distracted by the music. One thing I find difficult is when I *hear* myself breathing. I mentally tell myself that I am too tired to keep going. But if I can't hear myself breathe, I can keep going until my *body* tells me I am tired instead of my mind.

How many times has someone told you that you should take a picture of yourself and post it on your fridge or just weigh yourself every day or constantly monitor your calories as some sort of motivator to lose weight? Did they actually work at all? If they did work, then for how long?

The problem with seeking weight-loss advice or motivational tips is that people are generally looking outside themselves. In a nutshell, no one knows you like you know yourself, and obviously what worked for someone may not work for you. But what's most important is remembering that choices you make come from inside of you. No one else is telling you not to exercise and no one else is telling you to eat that brownie.

Pay attention to how food really affects you. A lot of people feel good when they eat junky, processed food but then immediately regret it after. Their feelings after they eat it are always the same: depression, guilt, and a hopelessness that no one should feel. Perhaps you felt a loss of willpower that unfortunately left you in a downward spiral.

Focus on what makes you feel good: eating nutritious food, getting your exercise in, and staying positive! Stick to a diet plan that is easy to follow and makes you feel alive and full of energy. Don't look for an easy way out to drop a few pounds. It takes discipline at first to get used to your new diet and healthy lifestyle. Always pay attention and listen to what your mind and body are really telling you.

Motivation is a key ingredient in any get-off-your-rear, take-action change in your life. Get focused on what you want out of life. Don't just say, "I want to be skinny." Being *healthy* is the most important goal. Being healthy will enable you to keep up with your kids—play with them and take them to all of their activities—and stop feeling like it is a job rather than a gift. Create lifelong memories with them. Think of them as part of your motivation.

Picture yourself every day the way you want to look. Visualize in your mind the type of life you would like to have. Meditate these visions and feelings into your everyday routine. List the things you are grateful for. Doing this now will help get rid of the negative feelings that bring us down. When we are down, we tend to give in to food since many of us turn to food as a crutch for happiness.

First thing in the morning, before you even get out of bed, visualize the new you, visualize yourself working out with more energy, and remind yourself of all you are grateful for. You will start your day on the right foot. If you start to get down on yourself and want to reach for unhealthy food, take a minute and really ask yourself why you are craving that right now. Try to determine if there is something that is triggering you to start overeating in the first place.

Getting to the root of the problem and dealing with it will help you free yourself of that burden that is driving you to overeat. There is always a reason that people let themselves lose control. Talk it out with a close friend or relative or anyone who can be supportive. Ask yourself, "What void do I have in my life that I am filling with unhealthy food?" Then visualize what you want to look and feel like and stick with it. You'll get back on track. You'll realize you really don't want that piece of cake after all. Remember, *being fit feels better than food tastes*. Repeat this saying to yourself every time you go to grab an unhealthy snack. Post it on your refrigerator to give you daily reminders.

Getting motivated takes some effort on your part. Subscribe to fitness magazines or read books that approach life in a positive way. Every bit of information you read will help. Other people's success stories are often big motivators. Once you add a workout routine and change your eating habits, your weight will just drop off—*if* you are consistent and stay with it. Eventually, it won't even feel like hard work; it will become a habit.

Just remember, do everything in moderation. You cannot put too much pressure on yourself. If you are taking in three to four thousand calories or more a day, it will be difficult for you to eat only 1,500 calories a day. But every day is a step toward the freedom you will feel when all that weight is gone.

Find things to give back to yourself. Make yourself feel good with things other than food. When you start to think and feel this way, you really will not depend on food so much. I cannot understand people who plan their next meal while they are still eating. That means you are using food as a means for entertainment. Food should be a source to fuel our bodies.

I know it is difficult in situations like parties or other social gatherings where the food is just staring you in the face. When you are in a crowd and everyone else is eating all of that fattening stuff, it feels like it is suddenly okay. You would be amazed how many calories you can add up with just a few bites. Remember that any drink, alcohol or not, can add up in calories as well. Be aware of everything you consume.

I see people ordering sugar-free tonic with vodka, but that is not calorie free! Don't fall for the sugar-free trap with alcohol. Alcohol will turn to sugar; if it is not burned off, it will then turn to fat. Everything we put in our mouths, whether it is fat free or sugar free, will turn to fat if it is not burned off before we go to bed.

Make your workout routine a priority. Set a schedule and stick with it. Think of your workouts as appointments that you *cannot* miss. I schedule everything around my workouts. I have my set schedule all week, and I try not to miss it for anything. I look forward to my workouts because I love the feeling I get when I am finished, and you will too. Stay with it; you will love yourself for it.

## Barbara's Tips for Staying Motivated

- Try to avoid being in situations where you will be pressured to "taste this" or where people might say, "One bite won't hurt you!"

- At parties, especially in the office, arrive with a cup of tea or coffee (or something similar) in your hand so your hands are full and you are not tempted to give in to temptation.

- Save the money on the packaged foods; buy fresh.

- Join a gym.

- Buy yourself new workout clothes. (This might motivate you to go to the gym so you can show them off!)

- Always eat before a party so you are full when you get there and won't be tempted by the finger foods that are loaded with calories!

# WHAT AND HOW TO EAT

As I started to work in my store helping people one on one with their meal plans, I was horrified to see how most people really eat. The sad truth is that our society has taught us to be so paranoid about everything we put in our mouths to a point where it is a detriment. People, especially women, do not eat nearly enough. Most are starving themselves to a point where they have symptoms of being mal-nourished! Ninety-five percent of the women I did diet plans for ate only two times a day. Most meals were not from the four food groups, not even close to being healthy! What these people did not know is that by starving yourself, you are only slowing your metabolism. Your next meal is only going to be stored as fat (no matter how healthy that meal might be!) because your body doesn't know when its next meal is coming, so it goes into survival mode! It is essential to feed your body properly at the right times with the right balanced foods. It is very important to eat protein with every meal. As long as you are feeding your muscle's protein, it will then force your body to use your stored fat as energy, which is your best source of energy!

We are living in a day and age where convenience outweighs the nutritional values of the foods we eat. Become an advocate of reading labels, and you will be amazed at how much crap you are unnecessarily putting into your system. It's no wonder we are fat and dying of terrible diseases. Use the clean food rule of thumb, which is do not eat anything that is processed or has preservatives in it, especially foods that have ingredients you cannot pronounce. When I know the source of everything that goes into my mouth, that is the type of food I call clean food.

It is amazing how unbelievable you will feel when you begin to eat this way. Limiting your sugar intake is important, and when you do so, you will have more energy than you ever knew you had! You will be able to exercise longer and more efficiently than ever. Your thoughts will be clearer and your moods stable. With all the foods today packed with sugars, fats, and preservatives, it is no wonder anti-depressants are one of the most prescribed medications in our country (Centers for Disease Control). Clean yourself out. You'll be amazed at how wonderful you'll feel inside and out.

Look in your pantry or refrigerator and begin to identify what foods contain ingredients you can't pronounce. I assure you, you'll find plenty! If you insist on using butter in your foods or if you're baking, use *real* butter, which is pure and natural. Margarine is a synthetic substitute for the natural thing.

Most people don't know the difference between the two. Both have the same amount of calories. Butter is slightly higher in saturated fats at 8 grams, compared to 5 grams for margarine. Margarine can increase heart disease in women by 53 percent over eating the same amount of butter, according to a recent Harvard medical study. Eating butter also increases the absorption of many other nutrients in other foods. Butter has many nutritional benefits where margarine has a few and only because they are added! Butter tastes much better than margarine, and it can enhance the flavors of other foods. If money is an issue, you will decrease your grocery bills by half if you buy all natural foods. What most of us don't realize is that we are paying for the packaging and convenience, not the food itself. (If you need convenience, follow the steps in the menu section to prepare your meals in advance.)

In the eighties, the buzz was that fat was the enemy. Later, carbohydrates were declared the enemy and fat became an ally. Do not follow the gimmicks to lose weight. The minute you stop dieting, the weight will come right back. Simply reducing fat is not enough either. It lures you into the illusion that it is okay to eat the whole box of low-fat cookies. The fat-free foods you choose may not have fat, but since they don't have fat, they are probably loaded with sugar to keep the taste. In reality, if you just ate the real thing (which you should allow yourself to do every once in a while), you would satisfy your craving. If you eat a whole box of low-fat cookies, I don't need to tell you how that would make you feel, not to mention you just ate a whole day's worth of calories on something that probably tasted like cardboard. Everything you eat that is not burned off turns into fat. It is so important not to get fooled by the fat-free claims! You have to watch out for these diet traps! That is why we need to change our *lifestyles,* not go on diets. Focus on the amount of consumption and the fats you eat.

Wheat breads can be another trap. Most people think that just because it's wheat, it's healthier. The truth is, in order for a bread to be able to claim it is a wheat bread, the manufacturers only have to add a small amount of wheat. Most likely, it still has the same ingredients as white bread. Most preservatives are not necessary, unless you plan to have the bread sit in your kitchen for a week or two.

In France, a country known for its bakeries, you will rarely see fat or overweight people. Why? They eat whole, real foods. They buy their bread fresh at the bakery, and it will last maybe two days. (I buy enough for two weeks and freeze it. I don't have time to go to the bakery every two days!) They buy their meat from the butcher and their fruits from the local outdoor markets. The key here is that nothing they eat has preservatives.

Preservatives are the problem in most people's diets, especially in our country. Eat what comes out of the ground or what you can prepare yourselves while at the same time enjoying the foods you love and controlling your weight. You will have more energy and look better, not to mention you'll be less prone to illness.

3. Foods made with white (processed) flour. Check the ingredients labels on breads, rolls, crackers, etc., and if the first ingredient says, "wheat flour," "enriched flour," or, "bleached flour," put it back on the shelf. The first ingredient should always be "whole wheat" or "whole grain" or another "whole" food. Try to avoid carbohydrates with dinner. This means no rice, pasta, potatoes, breads, or desserts. Carbohydrates at night only turn to sugar in your body. They don't have time to break down in your system before you go to bed. They sit there and turn to fat. Have you ever felt like you gained about five pounds overnight? Chances are you ate too many carbohydrates the night before. I guarantee that if you try not to eat any carbohydrates after 5:00 p.m., you will feel like you've lost five pounds the fol-

lowing day. If you keep doing this on a daily basis, you'll lose several pounds! It will become a habit. It's best to stick with a protein and a vegetable for dinner. Meal suggestions are in the menu section.

4.  Limit your fruit intake. Generally when people decide to lose weight, they run to the store to buy tons of fruits and vegetables. They swear they are going to eat like that forever. Guess which one they will eat all of? The fruit! Because it is packed with sugar. Sugar in your body will always turn to fat unless you burn it off, which most people don't. Stick with the vegetables! Give yourself a treat in the morning and eat a small amount of fruit with breakfast if you crave it. Try not to eat fruit after 12:00 p.m. If you eat it later than that, your body does not have the time to metabolize the sugar, and it will eventually turn to fat.

5. Unpronounceable ingredients. You know the labels that list ingredients that sound like something out of a chemistry experiment. The best foods to buy have the shortest ingredients list and have recognizable ingredients. Look for real food on the labels. My best source is saying to myself, "If God created it, it's safe to say we can eat it and stay healthy!"

Not eating enough, and at the wrong times, can make you fat. It is a fact that most people do not believe! Here are some examples of how this can happen and why it is so true!

Think of your body like a car that operates twenty-four hours a day. You would never expect your car to get you to one place or the other without refueling, just as you know you can't put more fuel than the tank of your car can hold. But why don't people see the needs of their own bodies as clearly as they see their cars? So many of us run on empty for hours and then end up adding more fuel into our systems than our bodies can handle. We would never do this to our cars, so why do we treat our bodies this way?

Let's say you really want to lose fat and lean out, so you decide to go for a run first thing in the morning on an empty stomach. The easiest way for your body to get energy is to break down muscle mass. The problem here is that by not eating before you go for that run, you are actually using that very same muscle you are trying to build on for energy. We need to build muscle in order to burn fat! The more muscle we have, the more fat we burn. We want to protect our muscles and build on them, not burn them and use them as energy. This process is called the muscle loss program; it's not good! Eat a small portion of carbs before that workout. Oatmeal is good or a half of a banana, just something small to give you the energy you need to get through your workout.

The most typical way people gain weight and never realize it is by waiting too long between meals.

Then when they do eat, they tend to overeat because they are so hungry. Not to mention that their bodies are in starvation mode, so it will hold onto anything that they put in because it has no idea when its next energy source is coming. It's your body's defense mechanism to keep you from starving. That means more fat storage! This is the fat gain program. Combine the two and you become a muscle-burning, fat-storage machine, something you do not want to become!

So many people live their lives this way, starving themselves and thinking they are doing the right thing to stay thin. They have no energy and feel that if they eat too often they will get fat. The opposite is true! You do not need to starve yourself to lose weight and be healthy! *Stop Dieting and Start Living!*

The way to get the perfect energy balance throughout the day is eating the right foods at the right times.

This means:

1. Eat as soon as you wake up in the morning. Have a time-released protein drink with a good glutamine peptide added to aggressively repair muscle.

2. Make sure you eat something small before you work out. If you don't, you will be burning the muscle you are trying to build.

3. Eat some kind of protein or have your protein shake with a Gluatmine peptide right after you work out. If you don't, your body will start burning muscle for energy.

4. Make sure you eat a protein, carb, and vegetable at every meal except your evening meal. (This should only consist of a protein and vegetable) Carbs will just turn to sugar if not burned off before you go to bed, and sugars turn to fat.

The worst strategy for losing weight is trying to starve yourself. Your metabolism will just shut down, and whatever you put in your body will then be stored as fat. Dramatically cutting calories will eventually result in weight gain.

Here is a good example of what a good eating plan should look like:

*(Times may vary)*

6:30 a.m.: Wake up. Immediately have a time-released protein shake with glutamine peptide, multivitamin.

9:30 a.m.: Eat a protein, carb, and vegetable

12:30 p.m.: Eat protein, carb, and vegetable

3:30 p.m.: Drink a protein shake with glutamine peptide

5:00 p.m.: Go to the gym: circuit training with weights

7:00 p.m.: (dinner) protein and vegetable (no carbs)

10:00 p.m.: (bedtime) protein shake with glutamine peptide

Here you have three meals with three added protein shakes. If you only ate the three meals listed above, you would burn muscle, not fat, which then leads to weight gain. When you add three time-released protein shakes, you are constantly feeding the muscle the protein it needs to build, which, in return, will burn the unwanted fat. So by adding the protein shakes and the added calories from the shakes, you will not be starving yourself and you will lose the weight. The normal body burns muscle while you sleep. By eating protein throughout the day, you are protecting and feeding that muscle day and night. It is so important that we build and protect our muscles as we age. We automatically lose muscle as we get older, so if we aim to build at a younger age, we will be better off when we are older.

If you follow the eating plan listed above, you don't have to restrict yourself from everything. You can have some flexibility and freedom to keep yourself from getting hungry and you will have the knowledge of knowing when and how to eat.

## Tips on how to stay on track:

- Focus on daily behavior as opposed to results.

- Drink at least one gallon of water per day. (Your body is 70 percent water).

- Prepare your meals ahead of time so they are ready to eat when you are hungry.

- Eat every three hours. (This keeps your metabolism going in order to burn fat and calories.)

- Eat before you get hungry. (This keeps you from overeating when you are hungry).

- No carbohydrates at dinner

- Eat at least one gram of protein per pound of lean body weight daily.

- Do thirty minutes of cardiovascular exercise four to five times per week.

- To figure heart rate zone for optimal fat burning:

  220–Age____=____X.75=____/6=
  beats per 10 second for heart rate zone.

- Work out with weights four to five times per week.

- Take one day off per week as your free day. (Rest and enjoy!)

- Take glutamine (preferably Peptide) with a time-released protein and a good multivitamin.

The following foods are some of the best foods to incorporate into your eating plan on a daily basis. These power foods added to your meals will not only satisfy your tastes and cravings but will help keep you from eating the dangerous fat promoters in your diet. Incorporate two or three of these foods into each of your three meals. Get a combination of protein, carbs, and vegetables in every meal (except in the evening). Make sure you get protein in every meal and snack.

Here are your best choices:

## Foods

Here are some of the best foods to incorporate into your daily plan.

### *Proteins*

*One serving equals the size of your flat hand*
> Chicken Breast
> Turkey Breast
> Lean Ground Turkey Breast
> Swordfish
> Orange Roughy
> Salmon
> Ahi Tuna
> Filet Mignon
> Cottage Cheese
> Top Round Steak
> Top Sirloin Steak
> Extra-Lean Ground Beef
> Tri-Tip Steak
> Egg Whites or Egg Substitutes

## *Carbohydrates*

*One serving equals the size of your clenched fist*

Fruit

Yams*

Sweet Potato*

Red Potato*

Steamed Brown Rice*

Steamed Wild Rice

Oatmeal*

Barley

Beans (Kidney, Pinto, Black)

Fat-Free Yogurt

Cream of Wheat

Squash

Whole Wheat Bread

Avoid flour products!

*Low glycemic carbohydrates

## Vegetables

*\*One serving equals as much as you want*

Broccoli

Asparagus

Romaine Lettuce

Green Beans

Cauliflower

Spinach

Green Peppers

Green Peas

Zucchini

Cucumber

Brussel Sprouts

Artichoke

Cabbage

No Corn

No Carrots

*Approved Condiments:* Spray butter, PAM, olive oil, Mrs. Dash, garlic powder, red or black pepper, mustard, salsa, low-sugar barbecue sauce, low-sodium soy sauce, balsamic vinaigrette, and Smart Beat mayo.

# Raw Nuts

- Build muscle, fights cravings
- Contain protein, monounsaturated fats, vitamin E, fiber, magnesium, folate, phosphorus
- Fight against obesity, heart disease, muscle loss, wrinkles, cancer, high blood pressure.
- Sidekicks: almonds, pumpkin seeds, sunflower seeds, avocados
- Nuts to avoid: roasted, salted, and smoked. Stick to only raw nuts!

Nuts are clearly out to help you. They are an easy, good-for-you snack at any time. They contain monounsaturated fats that clear your arteries and help you feel full.

All nuts are high in protein and monounsaturated fat. But almonds are the king of nuts. A handful of almonds provide half of the vitamin E you need in a day and 8 percent of the calcium. They also contain 19 percent of your daily requirements of magnesium, a key component for muscle building. In a Western Washington University study, people taking extra magnesium were able to lift 20 percent more weight and build more muscle than those who weren't. A Purdue University study showed that people who ate nuts high in monounsaturated fat felt full an hour and a half longer than those who ate fat-free foods like rice cakes, popcorn, etc.

# Beans and Legumes

- Build muscle, help burn fat, regulate digestion

- Contain added fiber, protein, iron, and folate

- Fight against obesity, colon cancer, heart disease, and high blood pressure.

- Sidekicks: lentils, peas, bean dips, hummus, edamame

- Beans to avoid: refried beans (high in saturated fats), baked beans (high in sugars)

Beans are good for your heart. The more you eat them, the more you'll be able to control your hunger. Beans are a low-calorie food packed with protein, fiber, and iron, ingredients crucial for building muscle and losing weight.

The best beans for your diet are:

 Soybeans

 Navy Beans

 Kidney Beans

 Pinto Beans

 Black Beans

 Lima Beans

 Garbanzo Beans

 White Kidney Beans

## Green Vegetables

- Neutralize free radicals, which are molecules that accelerate the aging process

- Super-food packed with vitamins including A, C and K, folate, minerals, including calcium and magnesium, fiber, and beta carotene.

- Fight against cancer, heart disease, stroke, obesity, and osteoporosis

- Sidekicks: spinach; broccoli; Brussels sprouts; green, yellow, red, and orange peppers; yellow beans; and asparagus.

Vegetables are packed with important nutrients, but they are also a critical part of your body-changing diet. Spinach is a favorite of mine because one serving supplies nearly a full day's supply of vitamin A and half of your vitamin C. It is also loaded with folate, a vitamin that protects against heart disease, stroke, and colon cancer. To incorporate it into your diet, you can use the fresh stuff as lettuce on a sandwich or in a salad.

Broccoli is another potent power vegetable. Its high in fiber and more densely packed with vitamins and minerals than almost any other food. It contains nearly 90 percent of the vitamin C of fresh orange juice and almost half as much calcium as milk. It is also a powerful defender against disease like cancer because it increases the enzymes that help detoxify carcinogens.

# Dairy

- Builds strong bones; fires up weight loss.

- Contains calcium, vitamins A and B12, riboflavin, phosphorus, potassium

- Fights against osteoporosis, obesity, high blood pressure, and cancer.

- Sidekicks: fat-free or low-fat milk, yogurt, cheese, and cottage cheese

Dairy gets so much attention for one thing it does well and that is strengthening the bones. It has other benefits as well. A University of Tennessee study found that dieters who consumed between 1,200 and 1,300 milligrams of calcium a day lost nearly twice as much weight as dieters getting less calcium. Researchers think that calcium probably prevents weight gain by increasing the breakdown of body fat and hampering its formation. Low-fat yogurt, cheeses, and other dairy products can play an important role in your diet.

# Oatmeal

- Boosts energy and sex drive, reduces cholesterol, maintains blood-sugar levels
- Contains complex carbohydrates and fiber
- Fights against heart disease, diabetes, colon cancer, obesity
- Sidekicks: high-fiber cereals like All Bran and Fiber One
- Stay away from cereals with added sugar and high-fructose corn syrup

Oatmeal contains soluble fiber, meaning that it attracts fluid and stays in your stomach longer than insoluble fiber (like vegetables).

Soluble fiber is thought to reduce blood cholesterol by binding with digestive acids made from cholesterol and sending them out of your body. When this happens, your liver has to pull cholesterol from your blood to make more digestive acids and your bad cholesterol levels drop.

Everyone needs more fiber. Doctors recommend we get between twenty-five and thirty-five grams of fiber per day, but most of us get half that. Fiber protects you from heart disease and colon cancer by sweeping carcinogens out of the intestines quickly.

A study at Penn State University showed that oatmeal sustains your blood sugar levels longer than many other foods, which keeps your insulin levels stable and ensures you won't be starving for the few hours that follow. That's good because spikes in the production of insulin slow your metabolism and send a signal to the body that it is time to start storing fat. Since oatmeal breaks down slowly in the stomach, it causes less of a spike in insulin levels than foods like bagels. Eat breakfast! A U.S. Navy study found that simply eating breakfast increased your metabolism by 10 percent.

# Eggs

- Build muscle, burn fat
- Contains protein, vitamin B12, vitamin A
- Fights against obesity

For a long time, eggs were considered evil and doctors were more likely to recommend staying away from them. This was all because they were known to be high in cholesterol. By tossing the yolk and eating the whites, you can reduce the cholesterol. More and more research shows that eating an egg or two a day will not raise your cholesterol levels as once previously believed. In fact, we've learned that most blood cholesterol is made by the body from dietary fat, not dietary cholesterol. That's why you should take advantage of eggs and their powerful makeup of protein. The protein in eggs is more effective in building muscle than proteins from other sources. Eggs contain vitamin B12, which is necessary for fat breakdown.

# Lean Meats

- Build muscle, improve immune system
- Contain protein, iron, zinc, creatine (beef), omega-3 fatty acids (fish)
- Vitamins B6 (chicken and fish), phosphorus, potassium
- Fight against obesity, various diseases
- Sidekicks: shellfish, Canadian bacon
- Stay away from sausage, bacon, cured meats, ham, fatty cuts of steak like T-bone and rib eye

It takes more energy to digest the protein in meat than it does to digest carbohydrates or fat, so the more protein you eat, the more calories you burn. Many studies support the notion that high-protein diets promote weight loss. Among meats, turkey breast is the leanest of meats you'll find, and it packs nearly one-third of your daily requirements of niacin and vitamin B6. Dark meat has lots of zinc and iron but tends to have more fat. Beef is a classic muscle-building protein. It's the top food source for creatine, the substance your body uses when you lift weights. Beef does contain saturated fats, so concentrate more on fish like tuna and salmon because they contain the healthy fats we need like omega-3 fatty acids as well as protein. Researchers in Stockholm studied the diets of more than six thousand men and found that those who ate no fish at all had three times the risk of prostate cancer than those who ate it regularly.

# Food Facts

## *Fats*

We all need *some* fat in our diets. Fat helps the nutrients get absorbed into our bodies. However, when consumed in excess, that amount of fat will contribute to significant weight gain, heart disease, strokes, and some types of cancers. There are two kinds of fats: the good and the bad. The key is to replace the bad with the good.

## *The Bad Fats (Healthcastle.Com)*

### Saturated Fat

These fats are mainly found in animal products, such as fatty red meats, dairy, and seafood. The oils that are marketed to be plant foods but are modified and enhanced by humans are coconut oil, palm kern oil, and palm oil. These are all bad for you.

## Trans Fat

Trans fats are invented, manmade fats and are also used as preservatives in foods to help prolong shelf life. Who wants to eat something that can last *years?* Did you know a Twinkie has the shelf life of twenty-plus years? It is scary to think that whatever is in these foods will stay *in our bodies* for that many years. We don't even know if our bodies can metabolize the ingredients in these foods. Think of the buildup of chemicals, toxins, etc., in our bodies. Once again, the fats we are talking about are more commonly known as partially hydrogenated oil. You can find this oil in 99 percent of all packaged foods, frozen or not. Most cookies, crackers, chips, fried foods, and the synthetic margarine spreads all have trans fat in them. We are all feeding these foods to our precious little children *and* ourselves. We would never want to hurt our kids, but some of the foods we are feeding them are so harmful. Stop now; save yourself and your children!

*The Good Fats*

### Monounsaturated Fat

Such fats include nuts, olive oil, avocado, and flax seed oil. These fats lower your cholesterol and increase the HDL, good cholesterol.

### Polyunsaturated Fat

This fat can be found in some fish as well as corn, soy, and sunflower oils. Omega-3 fatty acids also belong in this group.

## Supplements and Vitamins

According to recent studies, most people are lacking most vitamins needed on a daily basis. The best way to get these vitamins is from whole foods, yet most of us rarely do. For instance, we need fifteen milligrams of vitamin E a day to help protect against heart disease; it also helps build our immune systems. If your meals are low in fat, you are most likely vitamin E-deficient.

You can get vitamin E in naturally fat-rich foods such as nuts, seeds, olive oil, and avocados.

Proper amounts of iron are also essential. Iron helps deliver oxygen into our bloodstream. Once again, if you eliminate fats altogether, you might not get the iron you need, which is found in lean red meats like beef, lamb, pork, and poultry. If you choose to stay away from meats, you can also get iron from certain types of seafood such as oysters, clams, tuna, salmon, and shrimp. Iron is also found in dark green, leafy vegetables like broccoli, spinach, asparagus, parsley, and Swiss chard.

Most people consume less than half of the potassium needed per day. Potassium aids in muscle contraction and regulates fluids and mineral balance when you exercise. If you are low in potassium, you are not eating enough fruits and vegetables. Baked potatoes (plain!) are a great source of potassium. White beans and tomatoes are a good source as well. There are so many sports drinks that claim they have all the minerals and potassium you need, but these drinks are also filled with sugar and, in the end, have little nutritious value. The best way to get these minerals is from the foods we eat. When you exercise, you should only drink water. You will gain weight and added calories from flavored waters and sports drinks.

Water is so important to all of us! Certainly bottled water is a convenience that helps us stay hydrated while on the go. But put convenience aside; bottled water often starts out as tap water. In fact, did you know that bottled water is sometimes nothing more than purified tap water? Fortunately, the U.S. Food and Drug Administration (FDA) has strict labeling rules for bottled water, but it's up to you to learn the differences between various terms and what they mean. There are three major types of bottled water.

Purified water is water that has been produced by distillation, deionization, reverse osmosis, or other suitable processes. Purified water may also be referred to as demineralized water.

Spring water is water that flows naturally from the earth and is collected directly from its natural source.

Mineral water is spring water that contains dissolved minerals and other trace elements (at least 250 parts per million) that come directly from the source.

In general, safety standards for bottled water and tap water are the same, with a few exceptions. For example, because tap water may become contaminated with lead as it travels through pipes, the government limits the amount of lead in tap water to fifteen parts per billion, whereas the limit is set below five parts per billion for bottled water. Another major difference is that tap water is often fluoridated, but most bottled waters are not.

Most people can safely drink water directly from the tap. If you want to improve the taste of tap water, you can purchase a water-filtration pitcher, which reduces the amount of chlorine in the tap water. As I always advise, have water readily available to drink throughout the day to stay hydrated. People often mistake thirst for hunger pangs! If you stay properly hydrated, you will be able to differentiate the two!

Zinc helps regulate metabolism. The best sources of zinc include beef, lamb, pork, crabmeat, turkey, chicken, lobster, clams, and salmon.

Magnesium is essential for energy production and muscle function. You can find magnesium in some seafood. If you really do not care for seafood, try bran cereal, cooked spinach, or black beans. The key is to get your vitamins from whole foods; yet we rarely ever get the recommended daily allowance for most vitamins through food because most people don't eat properly.

Protein is one of the most important foods we need to reach our fitness and nutrition goals. I use Pro5 by NU-TEK They have developed what I feel is an incredible-tasting, most effective, sustained-release protein supplement I have ever used. *Pro5* is also enriched with branched-chain amino acids, glutamine peptide, as well as all the essential amino acids, which are absolutely necessary for maintaining lean muscle while simultaneously aiding in the elimination of body fat. I suggest mixing *Pro5* in water and taking it between meals as a snack, after you workout, and again before bed.

Another great product is Glutacor by Katalyst. Glutacor is an advanced-bonded, hydrolyzed, glutamine-based supplement comprised of the most potent forms of glutamine and immune-system-boosting agents available. I mix one scoop of this with every protein shake. This supplement is designed to enhance muscle recovery and reduce muscle wasting. This puts your body in a much better state for obtaining lean muscle and burning body fat.

My favorite multivitamin-based supplement is called Nature's Fuel by NU-TEK. This is a great-tasting, nutritionally potent daily formula comprised of vitamins, minerals, amino acids, antioxidants, greens, and immune-supporting nutrients. This quick-dissolving powder formula provides fast absorption for maximum effectiveness. I have more energy; it boosts my immune system, improves my everyday feeling of well-being, and supercharges my natural healthy metabolism. I either add it to my protein shake or just mix it in a few ounces of cold water. It's easier to just add them all together in one shake. I also add a Nutek brand of freeze-dried organic vegetables and fruits to my first shake every morning.

As mentioned briefly above, essential fats or good fats not only have a plethora of health benefits and help the body function more effectively, they can also help you lose weight. Essential fatty acids (EFAs) are classified as unsaturated fatty acids and are divided into monounsaturated (MUFA) and polyunsaturated fatty acids (PUFA). These fats are considered essential because the human body needs them to function properly and survive. Nature's EFA by NU-TEK is, in my opinion, the most complete, sophisticated blend of omega-3, 6, and 9 essential fatty acids available. (It is the only brand I can say that does not leave you with that awful fishy aftertaste!)

Scientific research has shown how important it is for people to consume omega-3, 6, and 9 essential fatty acids (EFAs) in their diet for overall health and well-being. A lack of EFAs (good fats) in your diet can cause everything from increased body fat, hardening of the arteries, abnormal blood clot formation, coronary heart disease, high cholesterol, high blood pressure, certain types of cancer, diabetes, and the list goes on.

Additional info on these products can be found at www.Nutrishopladeraranch.com

## Barbara's Tips for Avoiding Unhealthy Traps

- Cut back on saturated fats, red meat, and butter.

- Increase your intake of the good fats found in avocados, nuts, and fish oils, which studies have found to have a protective effect on the body.

- Drink plenty of water instead of juices.

- Bake bread. If you have to, buy a bread machine. Now, you are in control of what goes in the bread. Get creative;

you can add any variety of healthy foods in your bread, such as whole grains, flax seed, nuts, dried fruits—get creative!

- Make cookies with your family. Kids love this! I always add oatmeal, flax seeds, protein powder, or some kind of organic cereal to my cookies. The kids don't know the difference.

- Avoid packaged foods and the frozen food section of the grocery store altogether.

- Avoid fats, sugar, anything processed, or anything you cannot pronounce!

- *Eat* a piece of fruit instead of drinking it.

- Try a soda alternative. Use seltzer water and mix with any 100 percent pure natural juices.

- Eat as many vegetables you want.

- Prepare fresh vegetables and grill your own meats.

# HEALTHY EATING AND LIVING

Today we have a huge problem with obesity. We live in a fast-paced, on-the-go world that prevents us from eating as well as we might like. As sad as it is, a lot of people don't even know where to begin to change their eating habits. They are so accustomed to fast food, prepared food, and convenience food; they take the easy way out.

According to the Centers for Disease Control, our nation is becoming fatter and fatter, with one in three Americans suffering from obesity and 33 percent being unhealthy and overweight. Just observe the majority of people when you are at an airport, amusement park, or carnival, for example. I am always shocked to see the types of foods people eat and how overweight most of them are.

The annual health care cost of obesity in the U.S. has doubled in less than a decade and may be as high as 147 billion dollars a year says new government-sponsored research. The study was conducted by researchers at RTI International, the Agency for Healthcare Research and Quality, and the U.S. Centers for Disease Control and Prevention (CDC) and is published in the July 27, 2008, issue of the health policy journal *Health Affairs.* For the study, which was funded by the CDC Foundation, lead author Dr. Eric Finkelstein, director of RTI's Public Health Economics Program, and colleagues analyzed data from the 1998 and 2006 Medical Expenditure Panel Surveys. They found that:

In 1998 the medical costs of obesity in the US
were estimated at around 78.5 billion dollars
a year, half of which was financed by Medicare and Medicaid (government health insurance for seniors and families on low incomes).
Between 1998 and 2006, the prevalence of obesity in the US went up by 37 percent. This rise
in obesity prevalence added 40 billion dollars
to the annual healthcare bill for obesity. The
annual healthcare costs of obesity could be as
high as 147 billion dollars for 2008. Obesity
is now responsible for 9.1 percent of annual
medical costs compared with 6.5 percent in
1998. The medical costs for an obese person
are 42 percent higher than for a person of normal weight. This equates to an additional 1,429
dollars per year: the costs for an obese person
on Medicare are even greater. Much of the
additional Medicare cost for an obese person
are the result of the added prescription drug
benefit. Medicare prescription drug payments
for obese recipients are about 600 dollars a
year more than for normal weight recipients.
Obesity accounts for 8.5 percet of Medicare

expenditure, 11.8 percent of Medicaid expenditure, and 12.9 percent of private insurance expenditure. The authors defined obesity as having a body mass index, BMI, higher than 30. BMI is the ratio of a person's weight in kilos to the square of their height in metres.

Finkelstein told the press that "Although bariatric surgery and other treatments for obesity are increasing in popularity, in actuality these treatments remain rare."

"As a result, the medical costs attributable to obesity are almost entirely a result of costs generated from treating the diseases that obesity promotes," he added, suggesting that as long as obesity prevails to the extent that it does today, it will continue to be a significant burden on health care.

The statistics above clearly show that people do not care about their health and they eat only to satisfy themselves, not necessarily for nutritional reasons. This is why our kids are gaining weight at such rapid paces. They watch and copy everything we do as parents. Inactivity is a great problem in our society. With the video games and TV the kids watch today, it is no wonder they are so out of shape. Are you one of these people? If so, then make this change now. You can do it!

We often wonder why our health costs continue to rise and there seems to be no end in sight. Each year, more American children are killed as a result of obesity than of gun violence. Obese children suffer higher levels of depression than pediatric chemotherapy patients. They have a lower quality of life at five times the rate of non-obese children. Overweight children who develop Type 2 Diabetes may have heart attacks and need coronary bypass surgery before they reach thirty years old. If they live their entire lives obese, they will most likely die young of complications associated with obesity (National Center for Health Statistics).

Think about it. If you, as adults, are obese, or even just overweight, you are putting your children at risk of being without parents early in their lives.

You are also taking a risk of cutting your children's lives short. Remember, children learn from example.

One of the main problems is that parents do not know how to make healthy choices for themselves and their families. We are all misled by the confusing packaging and marketing that occur in the food industry. Many of these products are marketed toward children, from *flavored* oatmeal to *fruit* rolls or chocolate *energy bars.* After eating these foods, kids may struggle to accept other flavors, such as the bitter tastes of many green veggies. They won't develop the ability to appreciate and eat a variety of foods if all they are exposed to is sweet, processed food. Too much sugar at a young age can prevent their taste buds from maturing.

One of the biggest myths for young children is that fruit juice is a good choice for them. Kids can gain huge amounts of weight from this alone. Often the packaging shows pictures and names of fruits, but the products contain no fruit at all. The package might say "100% Fruit-*Flavored* Juice," when, in all reality, it has only 10 percent real fruit juice and is packed with high fructose sugars and dyes. Most people don't realize that "fruit drink" does not mean fruit *juice,* even if it has pictures of fresh fruit on the box. This is definitely not good for adults or children.

Some of the worst products (with very little fruit at all) are cereals and yogurts. Products display pictures of fresh fruit on their packaging. This is misleading to the parents who are trying to provide healthy choices for their children. Parents think cereal is a great way to start the day. The box says it has the goodness of fruit, but it has no fruit in it at all. The fruit colors you see do not come from fruit but are really red and blue dye colors in the cereal in the shapes of fruit. In conducting my research for this book, I read many articles that suggested that food dyes have been known to cause many diseases and problems in children.

· · · · · · · · · · · · · · · · · · · · · · · · · · · · · · · · · · · · ·

Let's talk about the fast food chains, which say they are providing healthier choices, but the food that they claim is healthy is still not that healthy at all. You order a salad, and it comes with a packet of dressing. When people don't understand portions and serving sizes, they may think that since it came with the salad, it must be the right amount *for* the salad, and they, therefore, use the whole packet of dressing. You might as well just eat that Big Mac because the fat and calories in your salad and all that dressing are probably higher than the hamburger itself. Ask yourself, is it really worth the calories you are taking in?

How many people can really walk into a fast food place and buy healthy food? I watched one day when we were on a road trip and had stopped in to use the bathroom. I was waiting for my kids, and I sat there listening to what people were ordering. They would order a fruit parfait with a cinnamon roll on the side, or that salad with a side of fries and a Diet Coke. Come on! Don't sabotage yourself. Don't even tempt yourself. Do you really need to go to a fast food restaurant?

It is important to sit down for every meal. Not just dinner, but every time you eat a meal. This will not only help you remember what you ate and when, but it makes it easier to control your portions. Sitting down for meals with your family is one of the greatest gifts you can give them. This is when everyone can open up and learn to communicate in a positive and supportive environment. If children grow up in secure and loving homes, they have better chances of not using food as a means to fill other voids in their lives.

The best advice my mom ever gave me when my kids were babies was, "Always make your children eat *whatever* you eat." So I took whatever I had made for dinner and put it all in the blender and gave it to my babies. They loved it! They never wanted that bland baby food again! Now my children will try anything. They actually will pick the fried stuff off certain foods, eat egg whites, and are not that into baked goods. I know this seems shocking, but they eat this way because I do. They are little sponges, watching and listening to everything we say and do.

Parents can help their children a great deal to prevent diseases later on in life. It's never too late to start; small changes in how we raise our kids today are believed to bring huge advantages later on in their lives.

When my oldest son was twelve months old, we were in a Mommy and Me class together. Every week they had a different topic of discussion for the new moms. There was one topic that startled me so much that it has stayed with me all of these years. The topic was nutrition, and what startled me were the things that our government actually approves for consumption that are known contributors to disease.

If you look at most foods geared toward children, you will find that nine times out of ten, partially hydrogenated fats are listed. This synthetic fat has to be one of the worst things for *anyone* to consume. The nutritionist speaking to us said there was a study done (remember, this was thirteen years ago; I am sure it is worse now) that reported that the typical body was not decomposing at the normal rate it had been twenty years before that. Basically, what she is saying is that we are filling ourselves with preservatives that our bodies cannot digest. These are toxins and chemicals that are building up over time and taking over our bodies. No wonder we are seeing so many new diseases pop up in our lifetime. It's time to make a change.

## Barbara's Tips for Healthy Family Living

- Make plans to have a family sports game.
- Take a walk every night after dinner together.
- Go on family bike rides.
- Buy plain, organic yogurt, and add your own mix-ins of honey or natural, fresh, or dried fruits and nuts instead of sugary cereals or fruit-filled yogurts.

- Make compromises with sugar and your kids. If you eliminate the sugary cereals altogether, it will just make them want it more. Let them have it, but only if they let you mix it with healthy whole grain cereals or oatmeal with no added sugar.

- Try to sit down for dinner with your family. It's a time when you can all connect and learn what everyone is doing in his or her daily life. It's the time when you only have healthy foods to offer! The kids will get used to it!

# KIDS AND EATING

As parents, we spend a lot of time talking to our kids about the dangers of drugs, alcohol, and cigarettes and the need for safety on the Internet. But obesity is clearly one of the biggest concerns in the United States today and poses dangerous consequences to our children's physical and emotional health. We can reverse this epidemic by creating healthy home environments and regularly talking with our kids about the importance of eating the right foods and regular physical activity. Set good examples for them by being the best you can be. They mimic everything we do. Especially have a good mind-set about weight. Do not ever put a child down because of what he or she is eating or how he or she looks. It is extremely damaging and will last a lifetime, as I clearly know! When I was really young, I was a chubby little girl. I had lots of friends and was really very happy. I had a friend who lived across the street from me. Every summer we took turns spending time at each other's houses. One day her mom was making sandwiches, and I asked if I could have one. Her response was, "You really don't need one."

I was so hurt by those words that they have stuck with me to this day. From that day on, I was so self-conscious of what others thought of me. I remember going home trying to hide my tears because I didn't want my family to know what she had said for fear of them teasing me more. Think about it; do you sometimes say things to your kids that can be damaging to them? Really be aware of these at all times. It will make a huge difference in their lives.

I struggled with weight and body image until I was in high school. I was always worried what people thought of me and that they were watching what I was eating. When I was little, I hid in the pantry to eat Oreos so no one would see me. Can anyone relate to that? I'm sure a lot of us can!

These kinds of memories stay with us and potentially shape the way we make food decisions well into adulthood. They can cause a person to eat for comfort or to hurry and eat as much as she can before someone sees her for fear of being judged. Emotional eating is when you eat in response to feelings rather than hunger, usually as a way to suppress or relieve negative emotions. Stress, anxiety, sadness, boredom, anger, loneliness, relationship problems, and poor self-esteem can trigger emotional eating. When emotions determine your eating habits rather than your stomach, it can quickly lead to overeating, weight gain, and guilt.

When I was modeling, I saw it all. There were girls who got into drugs just to lose weight. They got mixed up with the wrong people and destroyed their lives. I had roommates who made themselves throw up in the shower just so no one would hear them. Most girls smoked and drank to control their appetites. The crazy thing is, they all looked terrible anyway and they stopped working because they couldn't keep jobs. But I know why they were pushed to those extremes. I heard it all too often. "Your thighs are too fat, your eyes are not far enough apart, your butt is too big, you are too short, and your feet look too big."

What these people did not understand was that we were not mannequins; we were *people*. We were young, impressionable teenagers who wanted to be accepted; yet instead we were always told of our inadequacies.

This is what affects kids; just a few wrong words can destroy a child's life. Be careful what you say to children and how you say it when it comes to food.

It is important to realize the effects of a parent's comments and attitude toward the children regarding their eating habits and body image.

Parents who put too much emphasis on physical appearance can set the stage for eating disorders in their children. Critical comments, even joking around, can do damage that will take years to undo. Research suggests that daughters of mothers with eating disorders may be at a higher risk of developing eating disorders themselves than children of mothers with few food or weight issues. Children learn attitudes about dieting and their bodies through observation.

A spokesperson for the American Dietitians Association states, "When a mother is dissatisfied with her body and frequently diets, her daughter will learn to base her self-worth on her appearance."

Even small comments, such as making negative statements about your own bulging thighs or how excited you are that you lost a few pounds, can send the wrong message to your kids that being thin is ultra-important. We need to focus on our healthy eating and lifestyles so our children see the importance of that instead of trying to be perfect in one way or another.

Similarly, if parents absolutely will not allow their children to have specific foods, kids will definitely binge whenever they have a chance.

I had a friend when I was young whose parents would never allow her to have any sugar, sweets, or soda at all. So, as expected, when we were at other friends' houses and were offered treats, she went crazy. She wouldn't even play with us because she was too concerned about what she was going to be able to eat before she had to go home. I am not even sure she enjoyed it; she was just gorging.

When parents restrict their children to such extremes, they run higher risks of pushing their kids to become binge eaters. Binge eaters eat when they are not even hungry.

All of these behaviors can set the stage for eating disorders in the future. Eating disorders are real and treatable illnesses that can be the most difficult thing a family has to deal with and can even cause death in some serious cases. The main types of disorders are anorexia nervosa and bulimia nervosa.

Eating disorders usually develop during adolescence or in early adulthood. In some cases, they can also be found as early as childhood and as late as middle or late adulthood. They usually start with people who have low self-esteem. Eating disorders are their way of having control over something, especially if they live in controlling environments.

When children grow up in environments where they feel they have to be perfect in every way, those traits will follow them forever and damage them beyond belief. This includes their own body images of themselves. If we put too much pressure on our children to look the way we want them to look, it can create years of turmoil for children without them even knowing why.

The things we say and do leave lasting impressions on our children. If we put too much emphasis on food and weight, they will start to obsess and try to be what we want them to be. Every child wants to be accepted, especially by his or her parents, and children will do whatever it takes, even losing weight when they do not need to.

Teenagers especially are at the most difficult stage of their lives. All around them, they are reminded by the media that they have to be skinny or perfect to matter in life.

Guide your kids at a young age and teach them to have healthy body images of themselves, not to expect perfection, and to eat healthy for the sake of their minds, bodies, and spirits.

Because of the judgments I dealt with as a child, I still to this day struggle with my body image. I was just in Hawaii for a vacation with my family. We had a great time, except for the fact that I was worried about how I looked in my bikini and whether the family thought I had gained any weight since the last time they had seen me. I wasn't able to exercise as much as I usually do because I had broken my foot. So I stressed that I was going to be judged on how I looked. I am still young, and I have three kids and should be proud of how I look. I have nothing to be ashamed of, but still today I carry these thoughts around. All because of a few hurtful words a mother said to me. Think about this and be aware of your judgments to your kids and yourself.

We need to look at ourselves and be proud of who we are. In ten years, we will most likely look back and wish we looked like we do today. We are here today to enjoy the person we are right now. Let's not waste any more time wishing we could be those other people. Start to enjoy life; it has so much to offer us; love who you are right now.

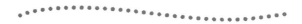

The first step to becoming a fit family centers on coming together as a family. It's incredibly important to have one central health message. If one child is overweight, it's crucial that you don't isolate that individual child. Instead, make this a project that benefits the entire family. Sit down together to discuss everyone's favorite foods and activities. Then come up with a family plan that incorporates everyone's ideas. If one kid likes pizza, plan a pizza-making night and supply them with only the best, healthiest ingredients. Use low-fat cheese, Turkey pepperoni, and lots of vegetables. This is not only fun for everyone, but they will take an interest in preparing food, which, in return, will make them more aware of good and bad choices. If another kid likes bike rides, plan a family outing with the entire family. A centralized goal of being healthy is good, but it doesn't need to be weight-loss specific. Once you have the whole family engaged in planning meals and activities, educating them about nutrition and fitness becomes easy.

Avoid eating meals in front of the TV. Kids in a University of Toronto study who ate in front of the TV consumed on average 228 more calories than those who didn't. If you are distracted during a meal, you'll enjoy your food less and lose track of how much you are eating, says Bonnies Taub-Dix, spokesperson for the American Dietetic Association.

Family-style eating is also not recommended. It is only going to make you fat. A serving of fluffy mashed potatoes on the table is just begging you to take a second or third helping. Instead, put a full portion on your plate at the beginning of the meal and leave the rest on the kitchen counter; you'll eat less. You will be surprised how little you need to feel satisfied. Another way to control portion size is once you have dished out the meal, put the leftovers away immediately before you sit down for dinner. This will prevent everyone from going back for seconds.

## Barbara's Tips for Keeping Kids Healthy

- Offer your kids vegetables with every meal. Keep trying. They will eventually begin to try them and like them.

- Do not ever be a slave or short-order cook to your children. They eat what *you* eat.

- Find a team sport for your children to join. It not only gives them the opportunity to exercise but also a chance to meet new and active friends!

- Encourage your kids to get outside. Don't let your children sit and watch TV or play video games while eating. This creates a habit of mindless eating; they will then start to eat out of habit and not hunger.

# GETTING STARTED

People start diets with expectations that are too high. I personally hate the word *diet*. Diet means temporary to me because with any diet, there is a start and there is an end. If you haven't learned the right tools to stay on track, you will go right back to your old ways. Once people reach their goal, if they ever even get there, they go back to how they were eating before, and guess what always happens? They gain it back with more to follow! We need to make *lifestyle* changes, not start diets. Make a choice to change your way of eating and lifestyle. With that will come a positive change in attitudes, appearance, and life! You really have to want it to reach your goals, so let's talk about how to get started.

Write a list of your healthy lifestyle questions. List as many answers as possible for each of these questions.

1.  Why do you want to get in physical shape?

2.  Why do you want to eat better?

3.  What types of motivation do you need to meet your goals?

4.  What types of exercising appeals to you?

5.  If you hate exercising, give yourself reasons why you think you hate it.

6.  Why does being healthy really matter to you?

Next to each answer, make two columns, one for the advantages and disadvantages of each. Answering these questions will give you a better idea of who you really are and how to help yourself get through the hardest time: the beginning. It should give you the motivation as well.

Buy a journal to list everything you put in your mouth and the time of day you eat. Document *everything*, even the crust off your child's sandwich! You will be amazed at how many extra calories you are eating without even noticing! Write down the foods you crave but can't have and make note of the time of day. There might be a pattern. (But try to hold back! The reward is coming!)

Figure out a time of day you can give yourself forty-five minutes to an hour of uninterrupted exercise. No answering the phone, doing chores, or stopping to accommodate kids. This is your time. Stick with this time. If something comes up, tell them you already have an appointment and cannot change it. Be firm! You are doing this for you!

- Go to the menu section of this book and make your grocery list.

- Buy yourself a new workout outfit or find something you feel good in while exercising.

Be proud of yourself for getting this far!

Before starting an exercise program, you need to understand all of the different aspects of it. The terms *exercise* and *physical activity* are often used interchangeably, but there are important distinctions between the two. Physical activity refers to any movement that involves muscle contractions and an increase in metabolism. This broad definition includes both aerobic and anaerobic activities. Types of physical activity are further divided into groupings based on the reasons a person performs the activity, such as transportation, recreation, or household chores.

If time is a concern, try choosing activities that are more vigorous and shorten the length of your workout. Just be sure that you don't have any health conditions that might make vigorous activity dangerous, and gradually work your way up to more intense exercise. Just your everyday chores can help. Household activities, such as sweeping or leisurely gardening, can be a good way to get moving. But there's no reason to stop there. Coupling this kind of activity with regular exercise will increase your total energy expenditure and improve your overall conditioning.

Knowing what you are striving for is a good way to begin. This knowledge will also come in handy down the road when you are setting goals, measuring your progress, and trying to get motivated.

What you eat and how you eat go hand in hand with your exercise program. It is important to eat something right when you wake up. If you are one of those people who can't eat breakfast, make a protein shake. You want to kick-start your metabolism. Drink eight ounces of water upon waking, and then eat every two and a half hours. Have your last meal about two hours before you go to bed. If you keep your meals small and the timing right, you will not starve between meals, which causes overeating when you do get to your next meal. (Do not skip meals.) Eating frequently also keeps your metabolism working constantly. Some people can last longer than three hours and some less than three. If you are not hungry after two and a half hours, just eat a small portion of protein. This will help your metabolism keep burning those unwanted calories. If you feel starved after only two hours, eat. Everyone's metabolism is different, so you'll need to see what works for you. The key is to keep making the right choices.

Frequent eating does not give you freedom to eat *whatever* you crave! You still need to choose the right meals and keep your portions small. This way of eating will also increase your energy to get you through the day. You will become a more efficient fat-burning machine. I often overhear people say to their trainers at the gym that they haven't eaten all day, as if it is supposed to be a good thing! What people do not realize is that the longer you wait between meals, the slower your metabolism will get! We have a built-in mechanism that protects us from starvation. Your metabolism will slow down because your body has no idea when the next meal will be. If you stick with it, you will get used to the proper way of eating, and it will soon be a habit. You will be able do this for the rest of your life and maintain the weight you have always wanted.

Change your life by changing your mind! Make it work for you by eating well-balanced meals and snacks. Make sure you confirm your cravings; a lot of people feel hungry when they are really just thirsty. Drink a glass of water before you eat and see if that takes care of the issue. Staying hydrated may also increase metabolism so you burn more fat. Keep water handy at all times, and drink all day long. Take a sip here and there; it adds up! Add a squeeze of lemon or lime juice to boost the flavor. These will also work as an antioxidant.

Visualize what you want and how you want to look. When we focus on the positives and look forward to something good, we take away the fear of failing. Don't tell yourself you have to lose a certain amount of weight or you are a failure. Tell yourself that you are going to be thinner in time and that making healthy choices and exercise are critical for your life. The more you say it, the more you are going to believe it and start living it.

Changing your way of thinking and your behavior toward food is going to be an ongoing process of staying aware and making the right choices. It will become a habit eventually and get easier when it starts to become your new way of life. But you need to train yourself and work at it; it won't come easily at first. So much of weight loss is in our heads. If your goals are too high, there is a sense that you cannot do it, and you will fail. Set yourself small goals, and reward yourself for each one. Ask yourself when you are reaching for that bag of chips or cookies, "Will that taste as good as being fit will feel?"

Believe it or not, family members and friends can make it difficult to eat healthy. Of course they love you, but they are used to your old way of life. It will take them time to adjust to the new, *healthy* you. Some people might even be envious of your choices because they have a hard time themselves. When you go out to dinner, don't let your friends give you a hard time for ordering healthy food. You don't need to worry about standing out or making them feel bad about their choices. It's not that difficult because most restaurants offer their main dishes as appetizers as well, which are in smaller portions. So order a dinner salad to start and an appetizer as your main course (with no bread, of course). If everyone wants a dessert (assuming there are six of you), suggest only ordering two for all of you to share, and choose to have only a little.

Alcohol is also a big contributor in calories without you even counting. If you go out for drinks with your friends, order a soda water to start. When you do order your drink, ask for water as well and alternate drinking them. Before you know it, it will be habit for you, and you still can be a part of the party. It is sad to say, but peer pressure can make you fat. Stand your ground, and hopefully your friends will pick up on your new great habits.

The reason so many diets programs fail is that people are not changing their lifestyles. Most of the weight-management companies out there sell you *their* food. You start to rely on these packaged foods, and the second you stop eating them, you will be lost regarding what to eat and how much. Really, how can you survive eating these meals forever? You won't know the right foods to eat or the portion sizes. The result after you have spent months showing up to these diet places, paying to be weighed, and buying the expensive food is *weight gain!* You might lose it while you are in the program, but you have not been taught the basics on how to live a healthy lifestyle forever!

Statistics (from the naturalcures.com Web site) show that most dieters are able to lose at least 10 percent of their total body weight as a result of dieting. Sixty-seven percent regain the weight they lost within a year after they stop dieting, and 95 percent regain the weight within five years. In addition, at least 33 percent end up gaining more weight than they had before they started the diet! The reason for this failure is simple. Diets do not teach you the balance or right lifestyle choices it takes to keep the weight off permanently. This makes perfect sense. It's an excellent marketing ploy. They want people to keep buying their products! Diets just don't work; there is a beginning and an end! So start living and stop dieting

Remember to keep that journal of every morsel you put in your mouth, and then try to calculate the calorie totals for each day. You will be alarmed in the beginning how much you ate that you were not aware of and also how fast the calories add up. You probably don't really crave or even want that little taste here and there; it is just a bad habit that needs to be broken. This is probably the worst habit a mother battles because she is constantly feeding her kids throughout the day. If you have this problem, chew gum when you make their meals and at cleanup time. You don't need to be eating the leftover food from their plates. Don't think of the wasted money; think of your health. Give yourself that long-needed attention you deserve.

Look at your workouts as an escape from reality. Save your best magazines to read on the treadmill. How many of you just sit and read these? Well, if you have time to sit and read a magazine or book, you sure do have time to work out! Once you get going, you will realize that it calms you down and releases that stress we all carry. You will then look forward to your time alone. So do yourself a favor. Work out!

# MENUS AND SHOPPING LIST

. . . . . . . . . . . . . . . . . . . . . . . . . . . . . . . . . . . . . .

Make sure you are feeding your body the nourishment it needs. That means getting it from the right foods! If you are not hungry at mealtime, only eat small portions. Listen to your body. Whenever I go out to dinner or eat at someone's house, I try to leave half of everything on my plate. That way I taste everything, and I won't offend anyone if the meal is not healthy. I can walk away feeling satisfied, not stuffed.

Try to eat upon waking to get your body going. The earlier, the better. Suppose you wake up at 7:00 a.m. Eat then. At about 9:30 a.m., have a snack; 12:00 p.m., lunch; 2:00 p.m., snack; 5:00 p.m., dinner; and 7:00 p.m., snack. You can obviously vary the times. Just try to keep the small meals about two or two and a half hours apart.

Here is an example of what a healthy day consists of:

6:45 a.m.: drink a protein shake mixed with a multivitamin powder (Nature's Fuel), fruits and greens (Nature's Fruits and Greens)

And take two EFAs (Essential Fatty Acids)

(Wake up kids; make lunches)

7:30 a.m.: take kids to school

8:00 a.m.: eat a bowl of oatmeal (not instant!), four fresh strawberries, six raw almonds

10:00 a.m.: go to the gym

11:30 a.m.: drink a protein shake

1:30 p.m.: eat chicken, brown rice, and broccoli

4:00 p.m.: eat about ten raw almonds, cottage cheese

7:00 p.m.: eat salmon with spinach, two EFAs

10:00 p.m.: drink a protein shake

10:15 p.m.: bedtime!

# Sample Breakfast Items

Any *one* of the following options will work for a healthy breakfast:

- 4 egg whites with one yolk for flavor (add as many vegetables as you like)

- 1 piece of toast with jam (If I am really craving bread, I'll have two pieces of whole grain bread bought from a bakery so it has no preservatives. I will not crave bread again all day.)

- 2 hardboiled eggs

- 1 cup of *nonfat* Greek yogurt. Add fresh berries or top with high-protein cereal (Nature's Best is a good example), or raw almonds

- 1 cup of high-protein cereal with light soy milk

- 1 cup of regular oatmeal with light soymilk, 1 tablespoon of raisins

- 1 slice of whole-wheat toast with 1 table-spoon peanut butter

- Coffee or tea with light soy milk (no sugar!)

- *Breakfast Burrito*

- Whole-wheat tortilla

- 4 scrambled eggs with one yolk

- Chopped tomatoes

- Fresh spinach

- Slice of avocado

- Salsa to taste

- *Protein Pancakes*

- 1 cup wheat flour

- 2 eggs

- 1/2 cup soy or nonfat milk

- 1 scoop protein powder

- 1/4 cup regular oatmeal

- Mix in fresh berries if desired.

- Cook as usual; the kids will not notice the difference!

## Morning Snacks

- Green apple with 1 tablespoon of organic peanut butter

- 1 bag of 98% fat-free popped popcorn (mini-size bag)

- 1 cup of fresh blueberries with 6 raw almonds

- Carrots or celery with 1 optional tablespoon of peanut butter

- One serving of Sugar-free Jell-O or pudding

- 1 plain, cooked chicken breast (just eat like an apple)

- Smoothie drink with ice, water, and frozen raspberries and any protein powder of your choice

# Lunch

- Dark lettuce salads like spinach or mixed baby greens. Avoid iceberg lettuce, which has no nutritional value at all. Do not add dressing or cheese. When eating out, ask for the dressing on the side. Good dressings to choose from would be balsamic, Italian, or olive oil and vinegar. My favorite is Girard's Light Champagne. Just dip your lettuce in the dressing. Do not drench your salad with it! People can actually gain weight eating salads. The dressing, lunchmeats, and cheese are the worst things you can add to a salad. Add tons of vegetables topped with grilled fish, chicken, and nuts instead

- Grilled chicken, fish, or flank steak

- Sushi is great, but limit the rice. Sashimi is best with little to no soy sauce. Eat as much edamame as you like! It is high in protein. Just make sure it is only lightly salted

- Soups with a water base are great, but no cream bases. They are too high in fat

- Ground turkey burgers topped with your favorite salsa, vegetables, and no bun

- Chicken breast with steamed vegetables and 1/2 cup of brown rice

- Turkey breast sliced and wrapped in a whole-wheat, low-fat tortilla filled with fresh spinach

## *Egg Salad*

4 hardboiled eggs (only use 2 yolks)

1 tablespoon of mustard

2 tablespoons nonfat yogurt

Salt and pepper to taste

Mix all ingredients together. Eat on a bed of dark green lettuce of your choice or one slice of whole grain bread

## Safe Pizza

Whole-wheat tortilla

Tomato sauce

Low-fat grated cheese

Turkey pepperoni

> Warm tortillas in pan, spread with tomato sauce, add cheese and pepperoni, and broil until cheese has melted.

## Tuna Salad

1 8-oz. can albacore tuna packed in water

1 tablespoon of mustard

> Mix together and serve with mixed greens and vegetables.

*For lunch, you can also choose from any dinners.

# Dinners

*Barbara's Chicken with Veggie Sauce*

4 boneless chicken breasts

2 cups chicken broth

3 fresh tomatoes

6 fresh basil leaves, chopped

10 mushrooms, chopped

1/2 cup baby carrots

1 zucchini

1 cup fresh spinach

> Sauté chicken in a pan sprayed with PAM nonstick spray. In separate pot, boil tomatoes, carrots, and zucchini in two cups chicken broth for ten minutes. Let cool for a few minutes and put in blender until a smooth sauce. Pour the sauce over the chicken and add the basil leaves, spinach, and mushrooms. Let simmer for ten minutes.

This sauce can be served over turkey meatballs as well. Use as a pasta sauce for kids who do not like vegetables! They will never know the difference!

### Zucchini Chicken Dinner

1 Boneless chicken breast

1 onion

2 cloves of garlic

2 cans stewed Italian blend tomatoes

1 basket of mushrooms, chopped

3 zucchinis, chopped

1/2 cup fresh basil, chopped

Brown chicken breasts in pan sprayed with PAM nonstick cooking spray; set aside. Brown onion and garlic. Add tomatoes, mushrooms, zucchini, and basil. Season with favorite spices; limit the salt. Add chicken and simmer for 1/2 hour.

*Grilled Flank Steak Dinner*

Approximately 16 oz. flank steak (4 oz. per person, serves 4)

1 basket mushrooms

1 onion

1 clove garlic

> Season meat and barbecue to your liking. In separate pan, sauté 1 basket of mushrooms with the chopped onion and 1 clove garlic in PAM non-stick cooking spray. Steam broccoli in separate pot, drain, and sprinkle with seasoning. Serve steak with a spoonful of mushrooms on top with the side of broccoli.

## *Grilled Salmon Salad Dinner*

4 4-oz. salmon filets

1 bunch spinach

3 hardboiled eggs

1 avocado

3 TBSP sunflower seeds

1 cucumber

2 tomatoes

6–8 leaves chopped, fresh basil

Fat-free raspberry dressing

> Season and grill salmon to your lik-
> ing. Toss remaining ingredients in large
> bowl and serve along with salmon.

## Chicken Tortilla Soup

4 cups low-sodium chicken broth

4 4-oz. chicken breasts

3 diced tomatoes

2 zucchini, chopped

1 onion, chopped

1 teaspoon cumin

Salt and pepper to taste

> Simmer all ingredients in a pot until the chicken is fully cooked; then shred the chicken to bite-sized pieces. Add sliced avocado and crumbled whole-grain tortilla chips for topping.

## Fresh Veggie Beef Soup

4 cups low-sodium chicken broth

10–12 oz. chopped flank steak

6 green onions

About 6 oz. bok choy, chopped

6–8 leaves chopped, fresh basil

½ cup chopped, fresh cilantro

2 chopped zucchini

1 basket sliced, fresh mushrooms

1 12-oz. can of stewed tomatoes

> Simmer all ingredients in a pot until the steak is fully cooked.

## *Pork Burritos*

6 pieces boneless pork chops (seasoned with salt and pepper)

4 cups low-sodium chicken broth

4 chopped tomatoes

1 chopped yellow onion, sautéed until brown

2 tablespoons cumin

1 teaspoon cayenne pepper

1 can green chilies

Boil pork in broth for 1 hour. Add tomatoes, onion, cumin, and cayenne pepper. Boil for 4 more hours or until meat falls apart. Add 1 can green chilies. Stir and serve with whole-wheat tortillas.

## Butternut Squash Soup

Bake a whole butternut squash in the oven at 350° until slightly golden. Let it cool and peel the skin off. Cut into small pieces and put in the blender or food processor until smooth. Add low-fat milk until desired soup texture and blend. Add 1 tablespoon of honey. Salt and pepper to taste.

## Garlic Rosemary Chicken

4 cloves of garlic, diced

1/2 yellow or white onions, chopped

6 boneless, skinless chicken breasts

1 cup chicken broth

1 zucchini, chopped

About 15 chopped mushrooms

3 tablespoons chopped rosemary

Sauté garlic and onions until golden brown in 1/2 tablespoon of olive oil or cooking spray. Remove from pan. In same pan, lightly brown 6 boneless, skinless chicken breasts. Add 1 cup of chicken broth. Add garlic and onions back to mixture and simmer for 20 minutes.

## Spicy Beef Stew

10–12 oz. lean beef, cut into cubes, lightly salted and peppered

1/2 chopped yellow or white onion

8 ounces peeled baby carrots

1 cup broccoli, cut into small pieces

2 teaspoons ground cumin

1 1/2 teaspoons pumpkin spice

1/2 teaspoon cayenne pepper

2 cups beef broth

> Sauté beef in 1/2 tablespoon of olive oil or cooking spray (about 2 minutes for medium rare). Remove from pan. Sauté vegetables together until golden brown. Add spices and broth. Add beef to mixture and simmer for 20 minutes.

> Buy small containers and fill with your own healthy satisfying foods. Just pop it in the microwave and you have your meal—just like you would those expensive, sodium-filled death traps they call a meal in a box. Save money and add years to your life and your family.

# Treats

## *Healthy Cookies*

Make the regular Nestle Toll House recipe but substitute with the following:

Use *whole wheat* flour, not white

Use *all brown sugar,* no white refined sugar

Use *real* butter, no margarine

Do not add salt

Add granola, flax seeds, protein powder, and/or *regular* oatmeal (not instant). Go to the bin section at your local health food store and be creative. Add as many healthy things as you like. Cookies are a great place to hide those healthy things we all need, especially for our children. Remember, this is still a *treat,* not an everyday food!

Sugar-free Jell-O

Sugar-free pudding

Sugar-free popsicles

# Shopping List

- ☐ Dark green leaf lettuce (no iceberg)
- ☐ Spinach
- ☐ Tomatoes
- ☐ Cucumbers
- ☐ Raw almonds/nuts
- ☐ Sunflower seeds
- ☐ Light balsamic dressing
- ☐ Dried cranberries
- ☐ Light champagne dressing
- ☐ Chicken breasts
- ☐ Fresh salmon
- ☐ Flank steak
- ☐ Pork chops
- ☐ Broccoli
- ☐ Green beans
- ☐ 98% fat-free popcorn (microwave in a bag)

- ☐ Organic peanut butter (pour 1/2 of the oil out before mixing)
- ☐ Light jam (not jelly)
- ☐ Tangerines
- ☐ Nonfat milk
- ☐ Organic light soy milk
- ☐ Nonfat Greek yogurt
- ☐ High-protein cereal
- ☐ Salt-free spices
- ☐ Protein powder
- ☐ Cliff Bars
- ☐ Lemons
- ☐ Bottled water
- ☐ Low-sodium sliced turkey breast
- ☐ Canned tuna
- ☐ Bagged spinach
- ☐ Sugar-free Jell-O

- ☐ Sugar-free pudding
- ☐ Zucchini
- ☐ Red onion
- ☐ Mushrooms
- ☐ Cherry tomatoes
- ☐ Brown rice
- ☐ Whole-wheat, whole-grain bread
- ☐ Eggs
- ☐ Fresh berries
- ☐ Avocados
- ☐ Ground turkey, 98 percent fat free
- ☐ Whole-wheat tortillas
- ☐ Tomato sauce
- ☐ Low-fat grated cheese
- ☐ Turkey pepperoni

# WORKING OUT

Exercise forty-five minutes to an hour every day. Walk, ride a bike, or go to your gym. Buy a fitness video if you have to. Just make sure you get at least forty-five minutes to an hour of activity a day. If you think about the span of an entire day, what is sixty minutes? It really is nothing to your day but does wonders for your mind and body. The more muscle you have, the more fat you will burn. Muscle becomes a fat-burning machine. Make sure you are eating enough, and do not skip meals. You want to get the most out of your workouts.

Everything has to come in moderation. I had a hard time with this one at first! Once I got pregnant, I thought it was a free-for-all regarding food. I saw food as a freebie: anything I wanted, any time I wanted—all rules went to the wind. I would be in bed at night eating a bowl of ice cream with my husband. I walked into the hospital to give birth fifty pounds later. I had a seven-pound baby, which is an average size, but not for a woman who gained fifty pounds. I was lucky he was healthy with no problems.

I later got pregnant again when my first baby was only six months old, which was a shock. I still had not lost all of the weight from the first pregnancy. I realized I had to be more careful how I ate this time around. I started eating the way I had before I had gotten pregnant. My second baby was eight pounds, and I only gained thirty-five pounds with him.

After that, I vowed I would never be overweight again. I started working out every single day. I lifted weights three times a week and did cardio seven days a week for one hour. I was obsessed. I ate very clean, maybe too much so, because I ate no fat at all. My body fat got down to 11 percent, which is very unhealthy for a woman. The average women's body fat percentage is about 20 to 25 percent.

It was so frustrating to the people around me. I never wanted to go out to dinner for fear of having to eat the butter they put on my vegetables and not knowing how they prepared my food. My family was not happy, and I was not living my life to the fullest. I got angry if I could not get my workouts in.

Then I got pregnant a third time when my second son was fifteen months old. This was a blessing in disguise. I was so worried that I would ruin my body since I had gotten it to perfection—so I thought. What I did not realize was that my insides were not perfect. I became constipated and moody, and my doctor kept telling me I was not gaining enough weight. I finally woke up and realized there is more to life than having a perfect body. I had a baby growing inside of me! I started working out three to four times a week. I ate healthy, but this time with the help of a nutritionist. I gained twenty-seven pounds with my third baby, and he was my biggest baby! Born two weeks early, he weighed eight and a half pounds. I had him in under two hours, and I lost the weight in one month by continuing to eat normally. This shows the power of healthy eating and exercise.

Today, I work out with weights four times a week and do cardio about four times a week. I feel great and have the energy to keep up with my three boys! The point I am making is that everything has to come in moderation. You need to stick with a program but not become obsessed or be lazy. Change your lifestyle.

Be a great role model for your kids. My boys see me work out all the time. My kids come to our home gym when I am in there and ask if they can work out too. How great is it that they really want to! They are always asking when they will be old enough to work out with Dad and me. So we have to come up with age-appropriate workouts for them. It is never too early to get your kids in the habit of exercising.

With any workout level listed, add any amount of cardio to your day if you want to challenge yourself. That also means to try not to get that parking place right in front. We all think we are so lucky when we find the coveted spot, but you really are not doing yourself a favor by being lazy. Look for the farthest spot and walk! Every little bit adds up, and it will help. Never take the elevator if you don't have to. Take the stairs! Constantly think of ways to challenge yourself. You can make a big difference with the little things you change in your everyday life.

Strength training, such as working out with weights or gym equipment that builds muscles, is very important for anybody trying to shed the pounds. Although aerobic exercises are most recommended for people who want to lose weight (and should definitely be a part of your workout routine), strength training is actually more effective at converting fat into lean muscle. Regular strength training also helps your body burn calories more efficiently for longer periods of time, improving your metabolic rates in the process.

While doing cardio, you are burning calories during your workout. While weight training, you will burn calories not only while you work out but for several hours after. Many women say they don't want to start weight training until they lose weight for fear of getting even bigger. The more muscle you have, the more fat you will burn. Start weight training along with cardio now. Besides, you are exercising not only to look your best, but, more importantly, for your health and wellness.

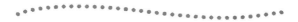

The following are sample weight-training workouts fit for the beginner (level 1), advanced (level 2), and experienced (level 3).

See the end of workout level 3 for pictures of each exercise performed.

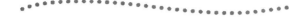

# Level 1

### *Monday and Friday:*

Warm up for five minutes walking on a treadmill, Stairmaster, or stationary bike. If you don't have access to this type of equipment, walk or jog outside.

### Bicep Curls

Sitting on the edge of a bench, use five-pound weights, keeping your body completely still, only moving your arms at the elbows, lift the weights up and down.

Do three sets of fifteen, resting for one minute between sets.

### Triceps

Holding a 2- to five-pound weight, standing with your knees slightly bent, bend over slightly and bring your arms to your sides. Only extend from your elbow down, holding the weights. You will feel this at the back of your upper arms.

Do three sets of fifteen, resting for one minute between sets.

## Back

Lie with your stomach facing down on a medicine ball and hold a five-pound weight in each hand, arms extended to each side. Bring arms down to the floor then out to your sides. You should feel this in your upper back.

Do three sets of fifteen, resting for one minute between sets.

## Shoulders

Standing with two- to five-pound weights in each hand, arms at your sides, legs slightly bent, bring your straight arms out to the side to shoulder height and back down again. Do not stop the movement to rest. This should be a constant motion.

Do three sets of fifteen, resting one minute between sets.

## Chest

Lie on your back on the medicine ball and hold five-pound weights in each hand, arms extended out. Bring straight arms together toward the ceiling.

Do three sets of fifteen, resting for one minute between sets.

### Ab Crunch on Ball

Sitting on the medicine ball with your lower back against the ball, arms folded, do crunches, making a full motion and bending all the way back until your head hits the ball and all the way forward so your arms touch your legs. Do this slowly and in control.

Do three sets of fifteen, resting one minute between sets.

## *Tuesday and Thursday:*

Do twenty minutes on an elliptical trainer and twenty minutes on treadmill, alternating walking and jogging. Jog for as long as you can. Stop and start as many times as needed. Just try to get some little bits of running in. If you don't have access to this type of equipment, walk or jog outside.

### Ab Crunch on Ball

Sitting on the medicine ball with your lower back against the ball, arms folded, do crunches, making a full motion and bending all the way back until your head hits the ball and all the way forward so your arms touch your legs. Do this slowly and in control.

Do three sets of fifteen, resting one minute between sets. Do your last set to fatigue.

## *Wednesday and Saturday:*

Warm up on an elliptical trainer, stationary bike, or treadmill for five minutes. If you don't have access to this type of equipment, walk or jog outside.

### Ball Squats

Get the medicine ball and put it against the wall. Lean against it with your lower back touching the ball. With five-pound weights in both hands and your feet apart, slightly pointing them out, squat down to a seated position. Do not stop at the top or bottom of this exercise. It should be done in a fluid motion.

Do three sets of fifteen, resting one minute between each set.

## Walking Lunges

Standing with five-pound weights in each hand, step forward and bend one knee at a time into a lunge position. Do not let your knee extend past your feet. You can really hurt your knees this way. Keep your upper body straight and abs tight.

Do three sets of fifteen on each leg. Rest one minute between sets.

## Side Leg Lifts

Lying on the ground on your side, lift your leg up toward the ceiling and then back down again. Do not let your leg rest at the bottom. This is one continuous motion.

Do three sets of fifteen on each leg. Rest one minute between sets.

### Back Leg Lifts

On your hands and knees, point your toe toward the ceiling. With your leg bent, lift your leg and do twenty-five reps on each leg.

Repeat this two times for each leg.

### Leg Extensions

Standing with one foot on a book or step, kick your free leg back, keeping it straight.

Do three sets of fifteen, resting one minute between sets.

### Cardio

Get back on a stationary bike, treadmill, or elliptical trainer for another twenty minutes. If you don't have access to this type of equipment, walk or jog outside.

### Ab Crunch on Ball

Sitting on the medicine ball with your lower back against the ball, arms folded, do crunches, making a full motion and bending all the way back until your head hits the ball and all the way forward so your arms touch your legs. Do this slowly and in control.

Do three sets of fifteen, resting thirty seconds between sets. Do your last set to fatigue.

### Sunday:

Off! Rest and eat well! This is your one cheat day. You get to eat *one* forbidden food item you craved this week. Try to eat only half of your normal portion.

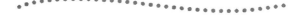

# Level 2

## *Monday and Friday:*

Warm up for fifteen minutes by walking or jogging on a treadmill, Stairmaster, or stationary bike. If you don't have access to this type of equipment, walk or jog outside.

### Bicep Curls

Sitting on the edge of a bench, use eight-pound weights, keeping body completely still and only moving your arms at the elbows lift the weights up and down.

Do three sets of fifteen, resting for thirty seconds between sets.

### Triceps

Holding a five-pound weight and standing with knees slightly bent, bend over slightly, and bring your arms to your sides. Only extend from your elbow down holding the weights. You will feel this at the back of your upper arms.

Do three sets of fifteen, resting for thirty seconds between sets.

### Hammer Curls

Standing with knees slightly bent and holding eight-pound dumbbells at your sides with the palms of your hands facing your body, bring weights up to your shoulders, bending at your elbows only.

Do three sets of fifteen.

### Tricep Dips

With your back facing a chair, grasp the front of the chair with forearms behind your back, feet forward. Bend slowly at your elbows, lowering your body to the floor. Then bring yourself back up to the starting position.

Do three sets of fifteen.

### Back

Lie with your stomach facing down on a medicine ball holding an eight-pound weight in each hand, arms extended to each side. Bring arms down to the floor then out to your sides. You should feel this in your upper back.

Do three sets of fifteen, resting for thirty seconds between sets.

### Shoulders

Standing with two- to five-pound weights in each hand, arms at your sides, legs slightly bent, bring your straight arms out to the side to shoulder height and back down again. Do not stop the movement to rest. This should be a constant motion.

Do three sets of fifteen, resting one minute between sets.

## Chest

Lie on your back on the medicine ball and hold eight-pound weights in each hand, arms extended out. Bring straight arms together toward the ceiling.

Do three sets of fifteen, resting for thirty seconds between sets.

## Shoulder Raises

Standing with legs slightly bent with five-pound dumbbells in each hand, keep both weights together at front. Raise weights in front of you, bending at the elbow and stopping when you get to shoulder height.

Do three sets of fifteen.

## Chair Push-Ups

With a chair or bench in front of you, place hands shoulder-width apart. Bend at the elbows, bringing your chest to the chair.

Do three sets of fifteen.

### Ab Crunch on Ball

Sitting on the medicine ball with your lower back against the ball, arms folded, do crunches, making a full motion and bending all the way back until your head hits the ball and all the way forward so your arms touch your legs. Do this slowly and in control.

Do four sets of twenty, resting one minute between sets. Do your last set to fatigue.

### Oblique Crunches

Lying on your side with your arms folded behind your neck and your knees bent, curl slightly up at the hips.

Do three sets of twenty.

Do some *cardio* of your choice for an additional fifteen minutes.

## *Tuesday and Thursday:*

### Cardio

Do twenty minutes on an elliptical trainer and twenty-five minutes on a treadmill, running most of the twenty-five minutes. If you don't have access to this type of equipment, walk or jog outside.

### Ab Crunch on Ball

Sitting on the medicine ball with your lower back against the ball, arms folded, do crunches, making a full motion and bending all the way back until your head hits the ball and all the way forward so your arms touch your legs. Do this slowly and in control.

Do four sets of twenty, resting thirty seconds between sets.

### Oblique Crunches

Lying on your side with your arms folded behind your neck and your knees bent, curl slightly up at the hips.

Do three sets of twenty.

## *Wednesday and Saturday:*

Warm up on an elliptical trainer, stationary bike, or treadmill for fifteen minutes. If you don't have access to this type of equipment, walk or jog outside.

### Ball Squats

Get the medicine ball, and put it against the wall. Lean against it with your lower back touching the ball. With eight-pound weights in both hands and your feet apart, slightly pointing out, squat down to a seated position. Do not stop at the top or bottom of this exercise. It should be done in a fluid motion.

Do three sets of fifteen, resting for thirty seconds between each set.

### Walking Lunges

Standing with five-pound weights in each hand, step forward and bend knee into a lunge position. Do not let your knee extend past your feet. You can really hurt your knees if your knee goes beyond your foot. Keep your upper body straight and abs tight.

Take twenty-five steps; repeat three times, resting for thirty seconds between sets.

## Side Leg Lifts

Lying on the ground on your side, lift your leg up toward the ceiling and then back down again. Do not let your leg rest at the bottom. This is one continuous motion.

Do three sets of twenty on each leg. Rest thirty seconds between sets.

## Back Leg Lifts

On your hands and knees, pointing your toe toward the ceiling, knees bent, lift your leg.

Do twenty-five reps on each leg. Repeat this four times for each leg.

## Leg Extensions

Standing with one foot on a book or step, kick your free leg back, keeping it straight.

Do three sets of fifteen, resting one minute between sets.

### Cardio

Get back on a stationary bike, treadmill, or elliptical trainer for another twenty minutes. If you don't have access to this type of equipment, walk or jog outside.

### Ab Crunch on Ball

Sitting on the medicine ball with your lower back against the ball, arms folded, do crunches, making a full motion and bending all the way back until your head hits the ball and all the way forward so your arms touch your legs. Do this slowly and in control.

Do four sets of twenty, resting thirty seconds between sets. Do your last set to fatigue.

### Oblique Crunches

Lying on your side with your arms folded behind your neck and your knees bent, curl slightly up at the hips.

Do three sets of twenty.

Do some *cardio* of your choice for an additional fifteen minutes.

## *Sunday:*

Off! Rest and eat well! This is your one cheat day. You get to eat *one* forbidden food item you craved this week. Try to eat only half of your normal portion.

# Level 3

*Monday and Friday:*

Warm up for fifteen minutes running on a tread-mill, Stairmaster, or stationary bike. If you don't have access to this type of equipment, walk or jog outside.

## Bicep Curls

Sitting on the edge of a bench, use ten- to fifteen-pound weights, keeping body completely still, only moving your arms at the elbows lift the weights up and down.

Do four sets of twenty, resting for thirty seconds between sets.

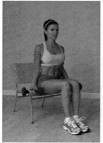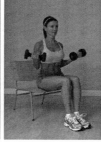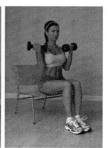

### Triceps

Holding an eight-pound weight and standing with your knees slightly bent, bend over slightly, and bring your arms to your sides. Only extend from your elbow down holding the weights. You will feel this at the back of your upper arms.

Do four sets of twenty, resting for thirty seconds between sets.

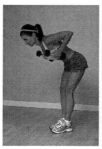 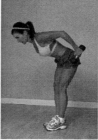 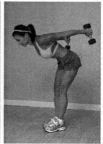

## Hammer Curls

Standing with your knees slightly bent, hold ten-to fifteen-pound dumbbells at your sides with the palms of your hands facing your body. Bring weights up to your shoulders, bending at your elbows only.

Do three sets of fifteen.

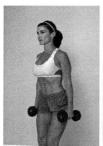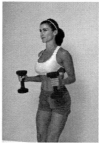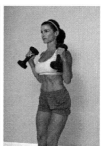

### Tricep Dips

With your back facing the chair, grasp the front of the chair with forearms behind your back, feet forward. Bend slowly at your elbows, lowering your body to the floor. Then bring yourself back up to starting position.

Do three sets of fifteen.

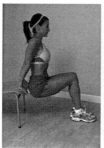 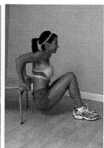

*More advanced version: put feet on the medicine ball and perform the dips as described above.

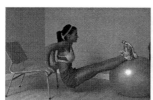 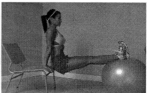

### Back

Lie on your stomach on a medicine ball, and hold five-to eight-pound weights in each hand, arms extended to each side. Bring arms down to the floor then out to your sides. You should feel this in your upper back.

Do four sets of twenty, resting for thirty seconds between sets.

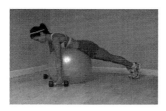

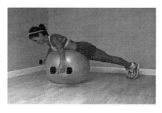

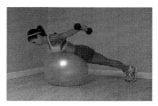

## Back

Bending your upper body forward with weights in each hand, lift to each side and back down to the front, as the picture shows.

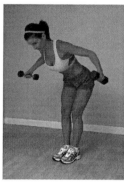 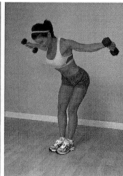

## Shoulders

Standing with five-pound weights in each hand, arms at your sides, legs slightly bent, bring your straight arms out to the side to shoulder height and back down again. Do not stop the movement to rest. This should be a constant motion.

Do three sets of fifteen, resting one minute between sets.

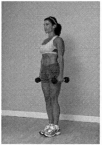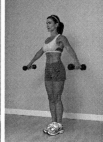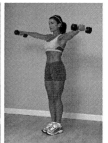

### Shoulders

In a sitting position, with your back supported on the chair, raise your arms up above your head and back down again.

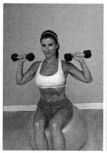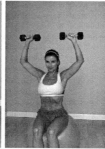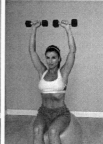

## Chest

Lie on your back on the medicine ball, holding ten-pound weights in each hand, arms extended out. Bring straight arms together toward the ceiling.

Do four sets of twenty, resting for thirty seconds between sets.

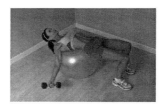

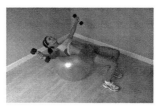

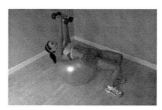

### Shoulder Raises

Standing with legs slightly bent, with five- to eight-pound dumbbells in each hand, keep both weights together at front. Raise weights in front of you, bending at the elbow and stopping when you get to shoulder height.

Do three sets of fifteen.

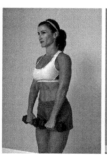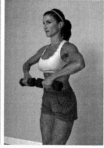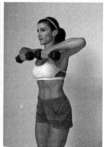

## Chair Push-Ups

With a chair or bench in front of you, place hands shoulder-width apart. Bend at the elbows, bringing your chest to the chair.

Do three sets of fifteen.

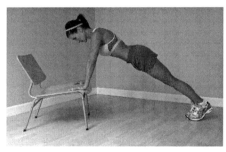

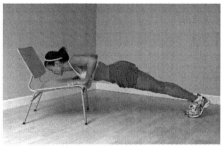

### Ab Crunch on Ball

Sitting on the medicine ball with your lower back against the ball and arms folded, do crunches, making a full motion and bending all the way back until your head hits the ball and all the way forward so your arms touch your legs. Do this slowly and in control.

Do eight sets of twenty-five, resting thirty seconds between sets.

Try to get two hundred sit ups every day. If it is too much all at once, do one hundred in the morning and one hundred in the evening before bed.

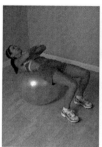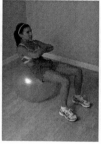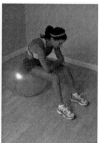

## Oblique Crunches

Lying on your side with your arms folded behind your neck and your knees bent, curl slightly up at the hips.

Do three sets of twenty.

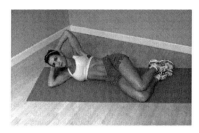

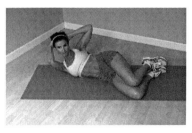

## Plank

Lie facedown on a mat, resting your weight on your elbows and keeping your feet straight out behind you. Keep your core tight and hold this position for the count of fifty.

Repeat three times.

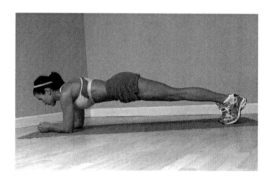

### Cardio

Do an additional fifteen minutes on an elliptical trainer, stationary bike, or treadmill. If you don't have access to this type of equipment, walk or jog outside.

## *Tuesday and Thursday:*

### Cardio

Do thirty minutes on an elliptical trainer and twenty minutes on a treadmill, running most of the twenty minutes. If you don't have access to this type of equipment, walk or jog outside.

### Ab Crunch on Ball

Sitting on the medicine ball with your lower back against the ball and arms folded, do crunches, making a full motion and bending all the way back until your head hits the ball and all the way forward so your arms touch your legs. Do this slowly and in control.

Do eight sets of twenty-five, resting thirty seconds between sets.

Try to get two hundred every day. If it is too much all at once, do one hundred in the morning and one hundred in the evening before bed.

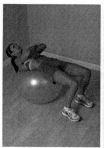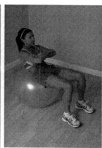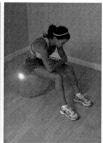

## Oblique Crunches

Lying on your side with your arms folded behind your
neck and your knees bent, curl slightly up at the hips.

Do three sets of twenty.

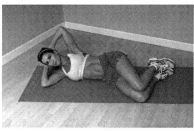

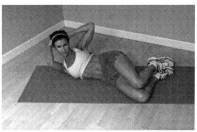

### Plank

Lie facedown on a mat, resting your weight on your elbows and keeping your feet straight out behind you. Keep your core tight and hold this position for the count of fifty.

Repeat three times.

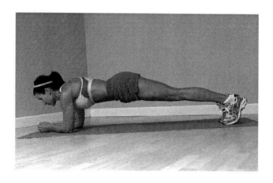

### *Wednesday and Saturday:*

Warm up for fifteen minutes walking on a tread-mill, Stairmaster, or stationary bike. If you don't have access to this type of equipment, walk or jog outside.

### Ball Squats

Get the medicine ball, and put it against the wall. Lean against it with your lower back touching the ball. With eight-pound weights in both hands and your feet apart, slightly pointing out, squat down to a seated position. Do not stop at the top or bottom of this exercise. It should be done in a fluid motion.

Do three sets of fifteen, resting thirty seconds between each set.

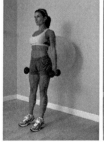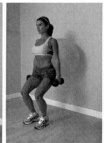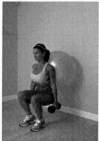

## Walking Lunges

Standing with five-pound weights in each hand, step forward and bend knee into a lunge position. Do not let your knee extend past your feet. You can really hurt your knees if your knee goes beyond your foot. Keep your upper body straight and abs tight.

Take twenty-five steps; repeat three times, resting thirty seconds between sets.

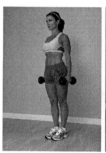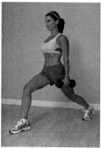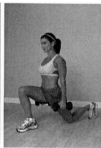

### Side Leg Lifts

Lying on the ground on your side, lift your leg up toward the ceiling and then back down again. Do not let your leg rest at the bottom. This is one continuous motion.

Do three sets of twenty on each leg.

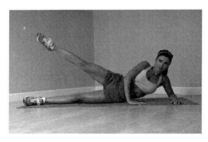

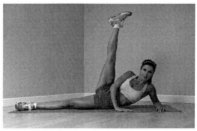

### Back Leg Lifts

On your hands and knees, point your toe toward the ceiling, with your knee bent and lift your leg.

Do twenty-five reps on each leg. Repeat this four times for each leg.

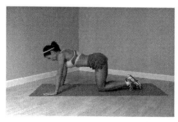

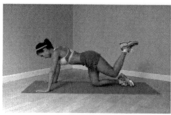

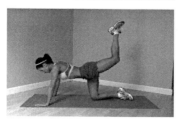

## Leg Extensions

Standing with one foot on a book or a step, kick your free leg back with your leg straight. Do three sets of twenty, resting thirty seconds between sets.

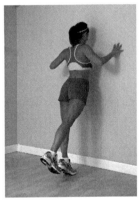 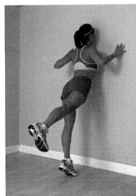

### Squats

While standing with feet slightly facing out and a little more than shoulder-width apart, hold a fifteen- to twenty-pound dumbbell with both hands in front of you. With your shoulders back and your back straight, squat down to a sitting position.

Do three sets of fifteen.

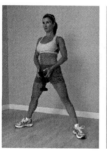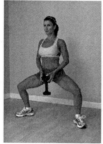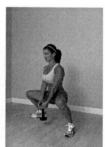

### Chair Step-Ups

With a chair or bench in front of you and your hands on your hips, step up with each leg twenty times and repeat each leg.

Do three sets.

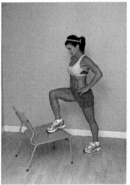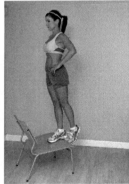

### Cardio

Get back on a stationary bike, treadmill, or elliptical trainer for another twenty minutes. If you don't have access to this type of equipment, walk or jog outside.

### Ab Crunch on Ball

Sitting on the medicine ball with your lower back against the ball and your arms folded, do crunches, making a full motion and bending all the way back until your head hits the ball and all the way forward so your arms touch your legs. Do this slowly and in control.

Do eight sets of twenty-five, resting thirty seconds between sets. Try to get two hundred every day. If it is too much all at once, do one hundred in the morning and one hundred in the evening before bed.

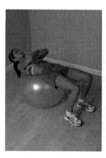 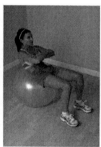 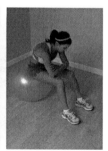

## Oblique Crunches

Lying on your side with your arms folded behind your neck and your knees bent, curl slightly up at the hips.

Do three sets of twenty.

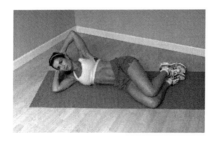

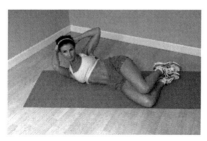

### Plank

Lie facedown on a mat, resting your weight on your elbows and keeping your feet straight out behind you. Keep your core tight, and hold this position for the count of fifty.

Repeat three times.

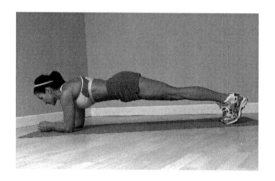

Do some *cardio* of your choice for an additional fifteen minutes.

## *Sunday:*

Off! Rest and eat well! This is your one cheat day. You get to eat *one* forbidden food item you craved this week. Try to eat only half of your normal portion. You'll even be surprised that you won't even feel like that dessert you craved all week!

If you can afford to do so, hire a certified personal trainer who can watch your form and change your workouts so you have a variety. If you can't, then get a friend you can count on and have the buddy system going. It's hard to flake out when you say you will be at the gym at a certain time and someone is counting on you. We are more likely to show up and lose the excuses when someone is waiting for us. Try to be consistent! You won't see results unless you work toward something.

# CONCLUSION

Congratulations! You did it! You are on your way to a healthier and happier life. Keep this little book handy at all times to be able to refer back and check your progress. It is hard to do this alone, so let me help by keeping you focused and motivated.

Change your lifestyle to fit the body you want and live that life. Whatever you visualize is what you create every day; visualize yourself at the weight you want to be. Tell yourself all of the great qualities you have. Write down all the reasons you deserve to be fit and healthy with an abundance of energy.

The impressions we make on our kids today can be damaging or healing for life. We need to find ways to help our children with good eating habits so they don't end up as overweight adults. Remember every day that our children are watching our every move. They will be affected by what we say to them.

Go to your pantry right now and throw away all of that crap that is sitting there waiting to cause damage. Do not think about the money you might be wasting. Think of how wonderful you are going to feel, how great you are going to look, and most of all, how healthy your entire family will be. Please do this for your kids and for yourself.

It all comes down to how you feel about yourself. If you are confident, healthy, and happy, your life can only be good. You can start now, at any age, to change your life forever. Do it now so you have more time on this earth to enjoy yourself and everyone around you. It is evident that more and more people make it a priority to start exercising when they start to get older. What a great accomplishment. You can achieve anything you put your mind to at any age!